This book is the coach you've been lookcal, doable map to declutter your home interior world so you experience the gi peace.

ANN VOSKAMP, author, *One Thousand Gifts*,
The Broken Way, and *WayMaker*

The Christian space has long needed a book like this—one that challenges the narrative of overconsumption while gently inviting us to examine the state of our inner world. Julia is a thought leader for the ages. She doesn't push or preach; instead, she shows up as a soothing presence who knows the way. This book is a brilliant blend of wisdom, practicality, and a profound call to declutter not just our surroundings but also our hearts and minds.

HANNAH BRENCHER, author, *The Unplugged Hours*
and *Come Matter Here*

Julia Ubbenga doesn't just teach you how to declutter your house—she shows you how to reclaim your peace, your purpose, and your connection with what matters most. Her honest storytelling, combined with practical tools, offers a lifeline to overwhelmed moms and anyone ready to let go of the noise and chaos of excess. This book is more than a guide to minimalism; it's an invitation to a freer, more joyful life.

ZOË KIM, author, *Minimalism for Families*

If you're looking for a guide to decluttering your stuff—not just your outer stuff but also your inner stuff—that leads to a lighter, more joy-filled life, then this is it! Julia's story serves as a powerful testimony that living with less can lead to a life rich in what truly matters.

ERICA LAYNE, bestselling author, *The Minimalist Way*

A profound and practical must-read! Julia understands that simplifying involves more than just decluttering our stuff—it also involves freeing our hearts, minds, and souls. Her personal story provides powerful inspiration to live a simple, more intentional life.

JOSHUA BECKER, founder, Becoming Minimalist

Julia invites readers to let go of their clutter and focus on what truly enriches their lives. In today's fast-paced world, this book provides a valuable guide to intentional and joyful living!

DIANE BODEN, creator and host, *Minimalist Moms Podcast*

Living in chaotic or cluttered spaces can do more than just make you feel overwhelmed or stressed; it can also affect your spiritual life. Julia does a remarkable job of showing you how to remove the mess not just within your home but also within your soul—so you can feel more present, less stressed, and further able to experience God's peace.

COURTNEY J. BURG, author, *Loyal to a Fault*

With *Declutter Your Heart and Your Home*, Julia's practical tools and thoughtful insights serve as evergreen reminders that minimalism is not only doable, it is also a lifestyle that directly reflects who we are and what matters most—living a joyful, intentional life.

CHRISTINE PLATT, author of bestseller
The Afrominimalist's Guide to Living with Less

Declutter Your Heart and Your Home is so needed in today's culture that tells us our worth is found in doing more, amassing more, and achieving more. Julia's personal stories and practical tools will help you clear your outer and inner stuff piles so you can more deeply enjoy your life.

DAWN MADSEN, founder, The Minimal Mom

In a world that constantly pulls us toward excess and distraction, Julia offers a refreshing and spiritually grounding perspective on minimalism. Our excess stuff clutters up more than the physical spaces within our homes; it clutters our minds and hearts as well. Julia does a masterful job of showing us how letting go of both the tangible and intangible clutter will leave us lighter, unhurried, less stressed, and free to pursue peace.

RACHELLE CRAWFORD, author, *Messy Minimalism*

Julia's passion for creating intentionally restful spaces for the soul shines through every page of this book. She beautifully demonstrates how to design peaceful environments that nurture both our mental and spiritual well-being. It's an absolute must-read for anyone who loves Christ and desires a clutter-free life anchored in him and focused on eternal things.

ANH LIN, author, *Forever Home* and
The Abundant Life Journal

Declutter Your Heart and Your Home is a breath of fresh air for anyone feeling overwhelmed by the clutter—both physical and mental—in their life. With warmth and wisdom, Julia invites readers to embrace simplicity and focus on what truly enriches their existence. In our fast-paced world, this is a powerful guide to living intentionally and finding joy in what matters most.

ANGEL CHERNOFF, *New York Times* bestselling
coauthor of *Getting Back to Happy*

Declutter Your Heart and Your Home

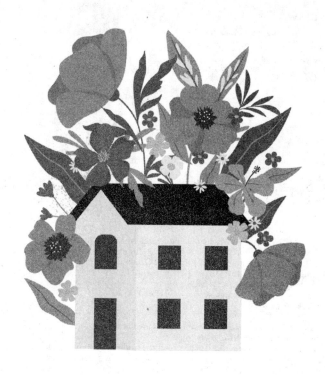

Declutter Your Heart and Your Home

HOW A MINIMALIST LIFE YIELDS MAXIMUM JOY

JULIA UBBENGA

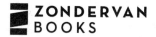

ZONDERVAN
BOOKS

ZONDERVAN BOOKS

Declutter Your Heart and Your Home
Copyright © 2025 by Julia Ubbenga

Published in Grand Rapids, Michigan, by Zondervan. Zondervan is a registered trademark of The Zondervan Corporation, L.L.C., a wholly owned subsidiary of HarperCollins Christian Publishing, Inc.

Requests for information should be addressed to customercare@harpercollins.com.

Zondervan titles may be purchased in bulk for educational, business, fundraising, or sales promotional use. For information, please email SpecialMarkets@Zondervan.com.

ISBN 978-0-310-36898-4 (audio)

Library of Congress Cataloging-in-Publication Data

Names: Ubbenga, Julia, 1984– author.
Title: Declutter your heart and your home : how a minimalist life yields maximum joy / Julia Ubbenga.
Description: Grand Rapids, Michigan : Zondervan Books, [2025]
Identifiers: LCCN 2024034826 (print) | LCCN 2024034827 (ebook) | ISBN 9780310368960 (trade paperback) | ISBN 9780310368977 (ebook)
Subjects: LCSH: Mothers—Religious life. | Motherhood—Religious aspects—Christianity. | BISAC: HOUSE & HOME / Cleaning, Caretaking & Organizing | RELIGION / Christian Living / Spiritual Growth
Classification: LCC BV4529.18 .U23 2025 (print) | LCC BV4529.18 (ebook) | DDC 248.8/431—dc23/eng/20240928
LC record available at https://lccn.loc.gov/2024034826
LC ebook record available at https://lccn.loc.gov/2024034827

Cover design: Lindy Kasler
Cover illustrations: Shutterstock
Interior design: Denise Froehlich

Printed in the United States of America

25 26 27 28 29 LBC 5 4 3 2 1

For my husband, Justin, and our children,
Eva, Elena, Ethan, Emelia,
and Evelyn
You make life rich

CONTENTS

PART 3: DECLUTTERING THE UPSTAIRS / MIND

INTRODUCTION

It was a Tuesday morning, nine o'clock. My back rested against the recliner chair, as I was too exhausted to feed the seven-month-old balanced on my lap.

Her big, expectant blue eyes locked on mine, triggering a wave of despondency in me.

Another thing to do.

I'd been working since 5:00 a.m. The work never stopped. When had life become a series of boxes to check off?

The baby's eyes shifted to my face. Chubby fists attached to my hair, pulling long strands as if to signal hunger.

I should have responded, but instead, my eyes scanned the room.

September sunlight filtered in through the window. I saw a Bible on the nightstand. An antidepressant prescription crumpled in a ball beside it. An unused crib filled to the brim with baby clothes, several pieces cascading onto the floor. Boxes of paper tottering high in a tower. Was that even safe? An assortment of plastic light-up toys, wrapping paper, and golf clubs.

All mine. Well, not technically all mine. But mine to care

for. The other rooms were no different. We had an endless influx of stuff.

A lot of stuff.

If these were my "best days," as my mom and mother-in-law had told me, I couldn't see it. I was blinded by a home stuffed to the seams with clutter.

I once read that the state of our home reflects the state of our soul. And so it was. Restlessness and angst, all on display.

The baby continued her attention-getting antics, blowing raspberries on my arm and then returning to hair pulling. A tight fistful and yank. Pain ensued.

Pain. I didn't even feel *that* much anymore. I'd leveled off at a perpetual state of numbness. Of doing. Of cleaning and organizing and fixing and buying. I was present but not present, there but not really there.

But I wanted to be there. To get back to the "me" beneath the outer and inner clutter. I wanted to enjoy my home and family.

To feel my soul again.

My exhaustion turned to anger. I thought of telling my hungry baby about it but decided that would be counterproductive. She wanted milk, not a revelation of my rock-bottom moment.

But I couldn't hold it in. My voice echoed against the beige nursery room walls.

"This isn't what I signed up for! What is really going on here?"

I realized I was talking to God.

"Something needs to change."

As if prompted, I reached for the Bible. I opened to the Gospels, and my eyes scanned the writings of Luke. A few minutes in, the words struck me, as if the answer to my aimless questions had been there all along.

- Your life does not consist of possessions. (Luke 12:15)
- Be rich in what matters. (Luke 12:21)

Rich in what matters.
Was *I* rich in what mattered?
The answer was no. A resounding, visceral no.
The words felt like a wake-up call. A call to live differently. To live a life of meaning, a life without regrets. A life without excess stuff.

I wasn't quite sure what it meant to become rich in what matters, but in that moment I resolved to find out. Because one thing felt clear: It was the path to getting my life back.

My rock-bottom moment in the nursery room recliner was five years ago. I'm a different person now. Transformed. Not at all who I used to be. Mainly, I attribute my change to a shift in three relationships: My relationship with stuff. My relationship with myself. And my relationship with God. The second two couldn't have happened without the first.

My relationship with stuff goes way back. I was born into a middle-class family with upper-class grandparents. My grandmother and grandfather had summer lake homes and winter homes on Arizona golf courses—not your typical couple. While my parents didn't shower me with stuff, my grandmother never missed a minute to display love through gift-giving. Sure, she gave the other twelve grandkids gifts too, but for some reason, she channeled the majority of her affection toward me.

One of my earliest memories involves three-year-old me hiding inside a clothing rack at a JCPenney department store, peering out and watching my grandmother shop. We shopped together often. Eventually, she'd realize I was missing and look distraught, so I'd jump out and scare her. She was never angry in her happy place. She'd be relieved to see me, pull me close, whisper, "You're my favorite, sweetheart," and then browse for something to buy me.

By the time I was six, she'd bought me everything from an expansive Cabbage Patch doll collection to a freckled hamster. Giving gifts was her love language, and I felt the love. I didn't often ask for more. I just happily received.

If this book had a photo section, I'd include one of me, age nine, with a wide buck-toothed grin, side ponytail, and tie-dye scrunchie, proudly sporting a T-shirt that reads "I Want What I Want When I Want It. Spoiled Brat." My grandma, who had gifted me the tee, stands beside me in our wallpapered living room. While *spoiled* usually holds a negative connotation, and *brat* most certainly does, if Grandma could have translated that shirt, I'm sure it would have read something like "I want what I want and I'm well loved."

When I was a teenager, Grandma and I would stroll Des Moines malls for hours, retiring only once the weight of the stuff-filled bags in our hands had nearly worn blisters on our palms. Gift-giving was her love language, and quality time is mine, so the hours spent filling those bags left both our hearts full.

Grandma was a great example in many ways. She modeled unceasing kindness and utmost respect for others. But through our years of shopping trips, I learned another important lesson—more stuff equals more happiness. Eventually, the "stuff + more stuff = happiness" equation became ingrained in me. Deeply. To the point where it was part of who I was. I didn't debate it or question it.

Grandma passed away a few months after I graduated from college. After she died, I was intent on filling the void and mitigating the pain, so I signed up for my first credit card and started buying. What my entry-level nine-to-five job couldn't cover, my credit card could. And once I realized I could spend on multiple cards at once, I began a collection.

Amassing stuff felt nostalgic. I'd spot items I knew Grandma would have wanted, like blazers or holiday-themed home decor, and I would linger in department stores, trying to catch a whiff of her favorite Elizabeth Taylor perfume. Buying also gave me a dopamine rush that I'd ride for a while, depending on the size of the purchase. But it never lasted, and soon I was left looking for more. As the saying goes, "You can never get enough of what you don't really need."

I'd become a cog stuck in the wheel of consumerism, and I was good at it. Make money, buy stuff, feel happy, feel restless, buy more stuff. Rinse. Repeat. At age twenty-five, I married my amazing husband, who didn't seem bothered by my spending. We went out to eat multiple times a week, filled our weekends with entertainment, and purchased what we wanted, when we wanted it. Our debt was growing, but life was good, as long as we could still put some money into savings and pay the minimums.

If this was adulting, we could play this game and win.

But we weren't winning. Not really. From the outside, our lives looked put together, but beneath the facade, we held our breath, hoping no unforeseen life event would unearth our "buy now, pay later" lifestyle. Our credit card debt soon topped $40,000. I tried to ignore it. When I did think of it, I felt bad, so I bought something new.

Soon the "shake-ups" came in waves: having a baby girl (high); not being able to afford a place to live after an out-of-state move (low); moving in with my parents (high); living there two years instead of the planned two months because of financial trouble (low); moving into a friend's rental home at a cut rate (high).

The feel of our new home soon bordered on claustrophobic and chaotic. Author Peter Walsh said, "Your home should be the antidote to stress, not the cause of it."[1] I agreed. I wanted home to be a restful, inviting place, and I figured it would be, as soon as I found the right stuff to fill it. So when I wasn't working my part-time speech-language pathologist job, I was out hunting for shiny new items to purchase at IKEA and Target.

I took both "jobs" seriously, and I wasn't home much. But my dream job was to be a stay-at-home mom. When our second daughter was born, my husband was promoted, and staying at home became an option. I was ecstatic.

My vision of stay-at-home mom life was idyllic. My daughters and I would be baking cookies, reading *Little House on the Prairie*, and giggling over tea parties. The transition was going great—until it wasn't.

Two weeks into the stay-at-home mom gig, I was less a

stay-at-home mom and more a full-time stuff manager. My days at home were inundated with picking things up, looking for things, tripping over things I hadn't yet picked up, and cleaning things. The life I'd imagined for our family soon felt inaccessible, hidden somewhere beneath our piles of possessions.

The people around me became moving "to-do" items, waiting to be checked off a list—feed them, bathe them, dress them . . . repeat—instead of people to enjoy. My stress level crept off the charts. My self-worth, often measured by achievement, was crumbling.

The clutter around and inside me continued to accumulate—an insidious filling of my home and soul. And now, both were nearing capacity.

As the levels of outer and inner clutter rose, there was nothing gradual about my feeling of numbness. It was a rapid onset, and three months after becoming a full-time stuff manager, I was diagnosed with postpartum depression.

An OB hastily handed me a Zoloft prescription, offering his condolences by saying, "If you were my wife, I'd want you to have this." It all felt odd. I opted against filling the prescription. How had life unraveled so fast?

Enter the rock-bottom, recliner-chair moment, when my words echoed off the nursery walls and I begged God to revive me. I had pleaded and God had promptly responded: "Your life does not consist of possessions. Be rich in what matters."

Now what? I had no idea.

Two days after this "possessions epiphany," I had a therapy appointment. I sat, perched on the therapist's sofa, baby Elena on my lap, overflowing diaper bag beside me. As the session came to an end, I placed the baby on my hip, heaved the bulky bag onto my back, and started toward the door.

"Julia," my therapist began thoughtfully, "have you ever heard of minimalism?"

Minimalism.

"You mean houses with white walls and next to nothing in them?" I replied.

The therapist smiled. "There's more to it than that. Look into it," she said. "I think you may be interested."

Look into minimalism.

I was intrigued. Sitting in my car immediately after the appointment, I did my first online search—keyword *minimalism*. A plethora of books, blogs, and podcasts popped onto my screen. Intrigue became interest, and soon I was hooked. I devoured all the resources I could find.

And then the aha moment happened: I didn't need all this stuff.

I didn't need it to be happier. I didn't need it to be liked, to have value, to look successful, or to give our children a good childhood.

Living with less stuff would mean more time and energy to focus on who and what mattered. Improved relationships, time immersed in prayer, space for a hobby I loved—it was all waiting for me there under the piles of random possessions. I didn't have to be a full-time stuff manager anymore.

I felt like a veil had been lifted. All along, the answer wasn't more. It was less.

I was still deeply entrenched in a tunnel of postpartum depression, but for the first time in months, I could envision an exit. Looking down that tunnel, I saw a small opening in the distance. With less stuff, I could fit through it.

Over the course of a year, 75 percent of our possessions went packing. With less stuff, I began to see that minimalism also applied to the "me" underneath my stuff. My inner clutter also needed to go.

As I jettisoned unneeded physical items, I realized I was curating two homes, an outer home and an inner home. The first housed my possessions; the second—the home of my soul—housed God.

In *Mere Christianity*, C. S. Lewis said,

> Imagine yourself as a living house, God comes in to rebuild. . . . At first, perhaps, you can understand what He is doing. He is getting the drains right and stopping the leaks in the roof and so on. . . . But presently He starts knocking the house about in a way that hurts abominably. . . . What on earth is He up to? The explanation is that He is building quite a different house from the one you thought of. . . . You thought you were being made into a decent little cottage: but He is building a palace. He intends to come and live in it Himself.[2]

God is ultimately what matters. And regardless of the state of our inner homes, he wants in. He wants space to rest and reside. He wants to guide us to a meaningful, rich, abundant life.

And it all starts with clearing the clutter.

Mother Teresa said, "The more you have, the more you are occupied. . . . But the less you have the more free you are."[3] True freedom is found in Jesus, and the less clutter you have distracting you externally and internally, the more time, energy, and attention you have to devote to life-giving union with him.

I've found this to be true. Instead of feeling numb, I now feel free to deeply experience and enjoy life. I'm no finished product—I'm still walking simplicity's path. So join me on this journey of physical and spiritual house-clearing.

As we go, we'll journey together through three sections of your outer and inner home and build the needed "toolbox" to declutter both:

Part 1: Laying the Foundation / Decluttering the Soul
Part 2: Decluttering the Main Floor / Heart
Part 3: Decluttering the Upstairs / Mind

Let's dive in.

PART 1

Laying the Foundation / Decluttering the Soul

Love the Lord your God with all your *heart* and with all your *soul* and with all your *mind*.

—JESUS (MATTHEW 23:37)

STRESSED OUT BY STUFF

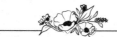

Every increased possession adds
increased anxiety onto our lives.

—RANDY ALCORN

The phrase *hot mess* joined our vernacular back in the 1800s to describe a warm meal, especially a gloopy one (think mess halls). This descriptor's most common target today? Moms. The term *hot mess mom* describes a person whose vocation is to care for little people but who does so in a chaotic state. In my experience, identifying with the "hot mess mom" label was driven by my internal state: I felt like I couldn't meet a set of self-conceived standards, so I gave up instead, and I rarely "had it together." If you google *hot mess mom*, descriptors include "disheveled appearance," "forgetful," and "unorganized." Parenting from a state of overwhelm has been normalized and even become expected.

Could the rise of moms who identify as a "hot mess" and the rise of stuff-ownership be related? Absolutely.

The average size of the American home has nearly tripled over the past fifty years.[1] In the 1950s, homes averaged 983 square feet. In 1970 the average home grew to 1,500 square feet, and in 2021 they averaged 2,480 square feet. And women's feelings of responsibility for home upkeep have persisted over those seven decades, according to a landmark study conducted by UCLA's Center on the Everyday Lives of Families (CELF).[2] Researchers studied the homes of thirty-two Los Angeles families over a period of four years (2001 to 2005) and published their findings in the book *Life at Home in the Twenty-First Century*. Having a larger home filled with more stuff, plus expectations to care for it all, is sure to unearth overwhelm. Every possession has a claim on the mother who cares for it. If considered clutter, these possessions constantly ping a mom's nervous system, activating fight-or-flight mode simply by being within eyesight.

Stress has become an epidemic.

We're living out a counterintuitive scatterplot: as the number of possessions has increased, happiness levels have decreased. You could debate causation versus correlation, but it still wouldn't change this fact: stuff-ownership is at an all-time high, while happiness levels are hitting record lows.

Data from the General Social Survey, which has been tracking Americans' happiness levels since 1972, indicates that 19 percent of Americans were "very happy" in 2022, which is the lowest number recorded in the past fifty years. Just a few years before, in 2018, the number of "very happy" Americans was 31 percent.[3]

Yet many of us continue to believe the lie that the more we have, the happier we'll be. The average US home now contains over 300,000 items, but 80 percent of the items people own are rarely used.[4] Fifty-four percent of Americans are overwhelmed by the amount of clutter they have, and 78 percent of those who call themselves overwhelmed report having no idea what to do with it.[5]

My own story reflects these trends. I didn't know it at the time, but in the metrics of happiness and possessions, my life was a microcosm of the culture at large. In accepting a life-draining, stuff-filled home, I accepted the low-grade stress that came with it. And in my surrender to this mindset, the door to my soul became stuck. Unable to open. Unable to receive God.

I swore by this more-stuff-equals-more-happiness mindset. And with each impulsive shopping trip I took, I taught this mindset to my daughter, just like my grandma had shared it with me.

Walmart became a "happy place" for Eva and me. We would go there multiple times a week, especially in the winter. I loved the light in her eyes upon surveying a new toy display. She'd engage with the toys, sometimes for up to an hour, while I watched or scrolled on my phone.

Walmart was where she learned to ride a bike. With a unicorn helmet on her head and a baby doll strapped to the bike of her choice, she'd cruise full loops around the bike display. We'd talk about going slow around the corners so as not to collide with an unsuspecting shopper. I thought I was instilling life lessons like respect and courtesy. More than anything, I was reinforcing our culture's lie that we can buy happiness. For me, for all of us, consumption itself isn't the problem— consumerism, or compulsory consumption, is. We all need basic things. But for many of us, our buying is based on what we've been told we need instead of what we actually need.

Joshua Fields Millburn of The Minimalists writes that compulsory consumerism rivals a prison, being "a voluntary incarceration," with us "caged by the invisible walls of consumption."[6] We're trapped within these walls. We know, deep down, that buying does nothing to placate our lack, but we know little else other than adhering to the norms of our consumer culture.

Too Much Stuff

The UCLA's CELF study,[7] mentioned previously, included dual-income, middle-class households with school-age children, representing a wide range of occupations and ethnic groups. The study generated almost 20,000 photos, 47 hours of family-narrated home video tours, and 1,540 hours of videotaped family interviews. Results confirmed one thing that virtually every middle-class American home has in common: a lot of stuff.

"For more than 40,000 years," write the authors, "intellectually modern humans have peopled the planet, but never before has any society accumulated so many personal possessions."[8]

Our society has accumulated the most possessions ever. Not only have we amassed a larger hoard than any culture through all of history, but this stuff-accumulation tendency has also become normalized. Even worse, it has become expected.

Researcher Elinor Ochs, linguistic anthropologist and

director of UCLA's CELF, explains, "What distinguishes us is the normative expectation of hyperconsumerism. American middle-class houses, especially in Los Angeles, are capacious; refrigerators are larger than elsewhere on the planet. Even so, we find food, toys and other purchases exceeding the confines of the home and overflowing into garages, piled up to the rafters with stockpiled extra stuff."[9]

Sound problematic? There's more. Besides confirming our stuff problem, researchers also investigated how clutter affects us.

Two of the CELF team's psychologists, Darby Saxbe and Rena Repetti, measured levels of cortisol (the stress hormone) in study participants' saliva. The researchers found that higher cortisol levels were more likely in moms who used words like "mess" and "very chaotic" to describe their homes and who had higher "stressful home scores." Lower cortisol levels were more likely in moms who had higher "restorative home scores."

Participants with higher cortisol levels maintained these higher levels throughout the day (instead of tapering off in the evening), leading to poorer sleep and increased anxiety.

We have more clutter than any generation in the history of the world, and this clutter is provoking a physiological response. We have created living environments that cause us to spend our days in a state of chronic stress. This leads to elevated anxiety, contributes to depression, and even reduces short-term memory. And yet we continue to accumulate.

In the words of comedian George Carlin, "A house is just a pile of stuff with a cover on it."[10] That covered stuff pile is doing more than just stressing us out. It's shaping our souls.

More Than Consumers

All this focus on stuff can alter our worldview, reduce our happiness, and misplace our identity. First, if we're not careful, materialism can indirectly distort the way we view others by leading us to prioritize possessions above people. A society founded on consumerism (continual buying and consuming of material possessions) can leave humans quickly devalued. Yet humans have eternal souls, and therefore infinite worth.

Archbishop Fulton Sheen said, "You must remember to love people and use things, rather than to love things and use people."[11]

But the ideology of loving things and using people is rampant. Roots often begin to grow in early childhood, as was the case with myself and my daughter. And then those roots become reinforced in our education system. "Here's a cursory vision of American education: we're teaching our children stuff, so that they can go do stuff, so that they can achieve and acquire stuff," said pastor Brian Schieber, "as if the whole point of life is to be this cog in a consumerist machine. And the goal of my life is to achieve material things so I can live a life of comfort. Is that really what we're made for? We're made for something greater; we're not just meant to be part of a consumerist machine. Our value isn't tied to what we produce or purchase. We have an inherent worth and dignity based on our very being."[12]

We are more than consumers. And when we weigh the value of a person based on extrinsic factors, we are, in a sense, dehumanizing them. A human is designed to make visible what is invisible: the spiritual and divine. To use the words of artist Bear Rinehart from my favorite band NEEDTOBREATHE's album *The Heat*, we are "signatures of the divine."[13] Not cogs in a consumerist machine.

The Gospel of America

Second, the gospel of America—the one that promises possession-based contentment—does not deliver happiness. The *actual* gospel does.

Jesus gives a road map to happiness in his Sermon on the Mount when he delivers the Beatitudes. His message is highly countercultural and contrary to America's "more stuff, more happiness" mantra. In the Beatitudes, Jesus shows us that happiness comes from God alone. He calls us to become poor in spirit, humbling ourselves, emptying ourselves, so as to be filled with him, not the things of the world.

The first beatitude, "Blessed are the poor in spirit," could be extended as an invitation to find happiness in a counter-cultural life:

> Blessed (happy) are you if you're not seeking happiness in the material things of the world. They are passing.
>
> Blessed (happy) are you if you're not chasing after the latest momentary feel-good high.
>
> Blessed (happy) are you if you're not addicted to the esteem of others and don't find your worth in their approval.
>
> Blessed (happy) are you if you are not making busyness an idol, rushing through this one life.

But we've bought America's gospel. A 2004 CNN poll asked Americans to identify the ingredients to happiness. Results included wealth, power, freedom from pain, positive self-esteem, honor, winning, and protecting our rights.[14] Emptying ourselves, becoming poor in spirit, and finding our identity in God? Nowhere on the list.

While we're busy filling our lives with the things of this world, God longs to fill every corner of our souls to the point of overflowing. To love us so much that it spills onto others. To be the companion who alone resides within our hearts. And he wants happiness for us.

Looking back now at my years of consumerism, I imagine God in a helicopter, hovering over my life, looking for a place to land, for time to spend with me, to imbue my life with happiness. But there wasn't space. The external and internal clutter left no landing site. He'd hover, come in close, catch my attention on occasion as the noisy rotary blades neared, but never land in my soul. Never stay and rest awhile.

Immersed in this stuff-centered, American gospel—wading blindly through a bog of inner and outer distraction and clutter—my life was full. Yet empty. Filled, but not with what mattered. Busy, but lacking connection with the one who mattered most: God.

As it turns out, the solution to uprooting our excess-induced stress and creating space for God is quite simple, albeit countercultural.

Inner Decluttering Tool: Find Your True Identity

Galatians states that our true identity is found as daughters and sons of Christ. "In Christ Jesus you are all children of God through faith, for all of you who were baptized into Christ have clothed yourselves with Christ" (Galatians 3:26–27). We are designed to find our identity in Christ, not from what we consume. But for many of us, things aren't just *things*; they are our identity.

Take time today to journal about your true identity. Consider the following questions:

- What does your mind gravitate to when you are asked to describe yourself?
- Are your descriptors primarily external, like your social status, your possessions, your profession, or your accomplishments?
- Or are they internal descriptors? Do you recognize that you are more than a consumer—you are a child of the Divine?

Summarize your true identity in a few words, then tape it to your bathroom mirror. Ask the Holy Spirit to etch this truth into your soul and to drown out any culturally imposed, false descriptors of yourself. When we realize we are children of God, we realize that "few things are needed—or indeed only one" (Luke 10:42). Soon our focus shifts away from accumulating stuff and back to the One who truly matters.

Outer Decluttering Tool: Get in Touch with Why You Buy

Living in a consumer culture, we're bombarded with advertisements and marketers' mind games, enticing us to buy. (Americans now see five thousand ads a day.)[15] It takes awareness and intentionality to be a conscious consumer, not a compulsive consumer.

To get in touch with why you buy, consider these questions:

- What drives your spending behavior?
- Are you buying to escape discontentment?
- Are you buying to uphold a certain image, thinking it will bring happiness?
- Are you buying out of boredom? Habit?

The field of psychology uses the acronym HALTS to describe states when we're more likely to act in an undesired way. HALTS stands for hungry, angry, lonely, tired, and sad/sick/stressed.

The next time you consider buying something, ask yourself, "If I weren't _____ (lonely, tired, sad, etc.), would I still buy this item?" If no, then don't buy it. If yes, then wait twenty-four hours before purchasing to see if you still need it.

CHAPTER

2

MINIMALISM: AN INVITATION TO FREEDOM

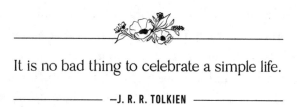

It is no bad thing to celebrate a simple life.

—J. R. R. TOLKIEN

It was Thursday, and I was on my way to the appointment where my therapist would invite me to look into minimalism. I had been mulling nonstop over the concept of life not being focused on possessions. I hadn't conjured up a road map or an ounce of guidance on how I was going to "arrive" at a simple life. The "less is more" idea was counterintuitive and in direct contrast to my worldview, but it was clearly what God was calling me to.

The baby, generally content on car rides, cooed from the back seat. As I shifted into the adjacent lane, her intonation rose with the car's movement. "She's happy we're going somewhere," I thought. "That we're moving forward."

Could I finally be moving forward? In contemplating simplicity, I started to see a way out of the perpetual grayness

13

that accompanied my life. The flame I'd felt enkindle burned faintly at the end of a long, dark path. Intuitively, I knew I needed to get there by refocusing and letting go.

"The point of simplicity is not efficiency, increased productivity or even living a healthier, more relaxed life," writes Jan Johnson in *Abundant Simplicity*. "The point is making space for treasuring God's own self."[1]

The call to a simple life was an invitation to freedom. To let go of everything that wasn't supporting me, serving me, or helping me build an outer and inner home centered on God.

I pulled our gold SUV onto the rocky driveway of the therapist's office, and then, heaving the baby, car seat, and diaper bag out of the cluttered car, I walked into the building where I would soon sit and disclose the workings of my inner home. My shoes crunched gravel. I realized I was holding my breath. I breathed and entered, oblivious that my next conversation would change the trajectory of my life.

"Julia, have you ever heard of minimalism?"

My therapist didn't elucidate, didn't expound, didn't preach the benefits of her questioning. She just waited. And then, as wise teachers do, she passed the onus onto me.

Through her questioning, my mind returned to the recliner-chair moment. I could describe the answer God handed me that September morning in many ways: guidance, a wake-up call, a subtle slap in the face, a paradigm shift, and an invitation to get my life back. The words I read in Luke stirred my soul, awakening something that stress and stuff had extinguished. It was as though the Holy Spirit, residing in the inner home of my soul, had rummaged through the overstuffed boxes, extracted a candle, and lit a tiny flame.

Your life does not consist of possessions. Be rich in what matters.

The pathway out of the stress-inducing, stuff-lined trenches—the pathway to a richer life—was *less*. My therapist's words had confirmed it. I knew, viscerally, that I was being called to a simpler life.

My Google searching began as soon as I returned to the car. Passing Cheerios into the back seat to appease the restless baby with one hand, I typed *minimalism* into my phone's search bar with the other and found an article by two guys who called themselves "The Minimalists."

"If we had to sum it up in a single sentence," they wrote, "we would say, *Minimalism is a tool to rid yourself of life's excess in favor of focusing on what's important—so you can find happiness, fulfillment, and freedom.*"[2]

True freedom, I knew, was found in Christ, in living in oneness with God. But my life was too cluttered for that. This idea of letting go of life's excess to find freedom and contentment in God sounded like an ancient practice applied to the material-obsessed Western world. Immediately, I liked it.

"Minimalism is a tool that can assist you in finding freedom," the authors continued. "Freedom from fear. Freedom from worry. Freedom from overwhelm. Freedom from guilt. Freedom from depression. Freedom from the trappings of the consumer culture we've built our lives around. Real freedom."[3]

I was burdened by every single one of these things. They weighed heavy on my soul—a soul that longed to feel light and free.

One of my favorite Bible verses is Galatians 5:1, where Paul writes, "It is for freedom that Christ has set us free. Stand firm, then, and do not let yourselves be burdened again by a yoke of slavery."

Another favorite is "Come to me, all you who are weary and burdened, and I will give you rest. Take my yoke upon you and learn from me, for I am gentle and humble in heart, and you will find rest for your souls. For my yoke is easy and my burden is light" (Matthew 11:28–30).

In the first century, a "yoke" referred to a rabbi's set of teachings on how to be human.[4] It was a rabbi's way of life, his method for "shouldering" the loads life brings. (Think of oxen yoked together to pull a cart.) Jesus invites us to a way of life that is unburdened, easy, and light, a way of life, or yoke, that is untethered and free.

Could a life of less stuff (inner and outer) be the light, easy, free way of life (yoke) I was looking for? Could simplicity free me from the burden of consumerism?

I was beginning to see the connection. In ridding myself of life's excess, I'd make space to apprentice under Jesus and find freedom. German theologian Eckhart von Hochheim's words, that "spirituality has much more to do with subtraction than it does with addition," suddenly made sense.[5]

If living rich in what mattered was the path God was calling me to walk, minimalism was my traveler's guide—my tool for the journey.

What Minimalism Is Not

The word *minimalism* has many connotations, not all of which are positive. It isn't about becoming like someone else—say, a perfectionist dressed in black whose modern home is always tidy because she owns only one hundred possessions and doesn't have kids. It's about becoming authentically you by clearing out clutter and aligning your life with your values.

While it does involve poverty of spirit—through humility and detachment, which I'll touch on later—minimalism isn't poverty itself. It isn't a home devoid of possessions or a set of rigid rules saying you can no longer enjoy material possessions. Minimalism isn't about living with *nothing*. It's about living with *less*. And if you're focused on owning a certain number of things, you're missing the point. (This one took me a while to learn—see the following section, "Minimalism as a Tool.") Minimalism looks different for everyone depending on their vocation and lifestyle. There is no minimalist mold to squeeze into, nor moral air about it.

Minimalism by itself isn't even a sure ticket to happiness. While minimalism will create space in your life, you still have to decide what to fill that space with. Getting rid of possessions will provide a dopamine rush (just like purchasing new possessions does), but it's temporary. Filling up that newfound space with something meaningful is what brings lasting joy.

Minimalism also isn't about organizing possessions. It isn't about spring cleaning, or rearranging the garage, or having a heyday with a label-making machine. It isn't about purchasing bins or packing possessions more efficiently into already purchased bins. It's about questioning the possessions that reside in your home and, if they aren't used or loved, letting them go. Minimalism is not organizing but de-owning.

At the end of the day, minimalism isn't really about your stuff at all. It's about the you underneath your stuff. It's about making space for our ever-present, ever-hovering God. It's about allowing him to land, take full residence in your decluttered inner home, and infuse authenticity, abundance, and meaning into your life by realigning your heart with what matters.

In the words of John Mark Comer, "The goal [of minimalism] isn't just to declutter your closet or garage, but to declutter your *life*. To clear away the myriad of distractions that rachet up our anxiety, feed us an endless stream of mind-numbing drivel, and anesthetize us to what really matters."[6]

Minimalism as a Tool

As I continued my journey, the lives of other minimalists soon became my fascination. I subscribed to blogs and podcasts, listened to audiobooks, marked the margins of paperback books, and even decided to start a blog myself, reawakening my love for writing. I called the blog *Rich in What Matters*, after the Bible verse in Luke that spoke to me, never imagining it would reach the eyes of millions of readers.

This modern movement toward simplicity (which I'd consider another term for minimalism) is nothing new, but rather a rediscovery of ancient spiritual practices.

Minimalism has its roots in the ancient world, but its core message—life is better with less—has been applied throughout the centuries. I read about the life of Socrates, who said, "The secret of happiness, you see, is not found in seeking more, but in developing the capacity to enjoy less."[7] I read about the lives of John the Baptist, Jesus, Mother Teresa, and Henry David Thoreau.

Reading about the lives of these minimalists—lives that left an indelible dent in world history—left me profoundly inspired but also, initially, off the mark. The goal of minimalism, I decided, was to own as little as possible—if Socrates didn't even own shoes, then surely I could do with only one pair. I began reading about modern-day minimalists who owned only one hundred things. Many lived a nomadic lifestyle, traveling the world with only the possessions on their back. While I hadn't yet begun decluttering, I had begun daydreaming.

"One hundred items—I wonder how close I am to that?" I thought. I held that number as the arbitrary guide rail to minimalism and decided that to *really* be living simply, my possession list would have to stay below it.

On a flight home from visiting family in Seattle, I began listing what I owned. By the time I got to possession number 323, the feeling of defeat was strong. With each addition to the list, my resolve to "go minimalist" dissipated a little more. 324: Hair dryer—oh, but I need that. 325: Blue scarf from Spain—oh, but I love that. 326: High school ring—oh, but aren't I supposed to own that? Every item I added felt painful. The "magic" number to achieve minimalist status felt well out of reach. I gave up making the list, considered burning it, and contemplated nixing the whole minimalism idea.

Right around the time I realized I'd had it all wrong, I settled on shredding the list. 327: Shredder—oh, just destroy the list already! Minimalism wasn't about some arbitrary set of rules. No one else could tell me what minimalism should look like for me. Sure, I could read about suggestions and guidelines, but ultimately, I was the one who would determine when I had "arrived" at a minimalist lifestyle.

To find inner and outer freedom, I had to embrace minimalism as a tool. That's what minimalism had been for everyone from Socrates to Mother Teresa—a means of supporting a laser-focused mission. These historical figures each had a clear and lucid "why" for living with less stuff. To amass more, they realized, would distract them from what truly mattered.

So, I wondered, what was my "why" for going minimalist? Once a minimalist, what would my mission-centered bio look like? "In 2018 as an overwhelmed mom of two, Julia let go of well over half her possessions and—" What? What was the purpose of this letting go? It wouldn't say "walked the outskirts of Kansas City barefoot." I had daughters to raise. It wouldn't say "entered a life of solitude living in a hut in a nearby Kansas prairie." I had a husband I loved and a house to care for.

In my asking these questions, the idea of minimalism was already calling me to identify my life's mission and purpose. What did I want my time on earth to look like? It was a question I'd never fully entertained when focusing on my next purchase or material acquisition.

In contemplating a rich life, what I was really asking was, What (and who) matters more than all this inner and outer clutter? In *The Power of Less*, author Leo Babauta writes, "Simplicity boils down to two steps: 1. Identify the essential. 2. Eliminate the rest."[8]

For me, "the essential" was relationships. What mattered

most was my relationship with my family, with myself, and above all, with God.

The Benefits of Minimalism

While the ultimate purpose of minimalism is to enter deeper into transformative union with God by making space for the Holy Spirit to reside in your inner home, many other "wins" arise along the journey to a simple life. I've had many aha moments, epiphanies if you will, while exploring why less is truly more.

In *The More of Less*, Joshua Becker speaks of the universal benefits of minimalism. "Excess possessions have the power to enslave us physically, psychologically, and financially," he writes. "Stuff is cumbersome and difficult to transport. It weighs on the spirit and makes us feel heavy. On the other hand, every time we remove an unnecessary item, we gain back a little freedom."[9]

If you're overwhelmed by clutter, then this "enslaved by stuff" metaphor likely resonates. It resonated deeply with me. Excess stuff weighed on my spirit. Life felt anything but light. I finally went all in on minimalism when I realized it was the most life-giving decision I could make.

Here are twenty reasons living with less stuff will also be life-giving for you, half of them inspired by Becker's *The More of Less*:[10]

1. **MORE PRESENCE.** With less stuff vying for our attention and devotion, we increase our capacity to show up fully present to the people we love.

2. **LESS WORRY.** If your time, energy, and attention are consumed by your possessions, then that's what you worry about. Every possession you accumulate adds another layer of anxiety to your life, while every possession you let go of is one less thing to concern yourself with.

3. **MORE CREATIVITY.** Owning less stuff results in a freer schedule with more margin to create and more mental capacity for creative plunges.

4. **MORE MONEY.** When you buy less stuff, more money stays in your bank account. Wanting less leads to consuming more mindfully and living within your budget.

5. **LESS STRESS.** An uncluttered environment means lower cortisol levels and less stress. Each additional possession we acquire increases the worry and stress in our lives.

6. **A DEEPER UNDERSTANDING OF YOUR AUTHENTIC SELF.** Owning less means having fewer culturally influenced purchases to hide behind. When these facades are cleared away, an authentic life emerges.

7. **MORE TIME AND ENERGY.** When you embrace a minimalist lifestyle, you have less stuff to clean and maintain. This equals more time and energy to allocate toward what matters.

8. **A BETTER EXAMPLE FOR YOUR CHILD.** Living with less shows your children that the most important things in life aren't actually things.

9. **LESS BUSYNESS.** A life with less stuff facilitates slower living. When you realize your home doesn't need to be overflowing, you realize your schedule would also benefit from more breathing room.

10. **MORE TRAVEL.** Owning less stuff means easier packing and increased ease of mobility. Moving houses is a less daunting task, and travel adventures are easier to pursue.

11. **MORE FREEDOM.** When you're not enslaved by your stuff, you feel freer mentally, physically, financially, and emotionally.

12. **MORE CONTENTMENT.** Having fewer possessions means having more space to discover what makes you deeply happy. Plus, when you stop using shopping to cover up hard feelings, you gain clarity on the true sources of discontentment in your life and can pursue healing.

13. **A DEEPER RELATIONSHIP WITH GOD.** Owning less means having more time to spend with God and fewer attachments. When consumer-driven distractions cease, your mind and heart become more available to God.

14. **LESS DISTRACTION.** Environmental clutter derails our attention; a clutter-free space facilitates increased focus.

15. **A BETTER UNDERSTANDING OF WHAT MATTERS.** When you eliminate the nonessentials, your values become clear, your actions align with them, and life becomes much richer for it.

16. **LESS ENVIRONMENTAL IMPACT.** Consuming less means causing less damage to our environment (and less demand for products unethically produced overseas).

17. **MORE GENEROSITY.** When you're not attached to your possessions, you're more able to bless others. More money in your bank account means more funds to donate to causes you're passionate about.

18. **LESS RESENTMENT.** With laser-like focus on what truly matters, you're more able to let go of petty things that don't. When letting go of stuff becomes your default mode, it's easier to do the same with grudges.

19. **LESS COMPARISON.** When you live with less, you embrace things that support your best life and you realize you don't need what others have to be happy.

20. **LESS DECISION FATIGUE.** Owning fewer possessions results in fewer choices (for example, deciding what to wear every morning). Studies show we have a limited amount of decision-making power each day. With less stuff, you minimize trivial decisions and save your mental energy for bigger decisions that matter.

By going all in on minimalism, Becker suggests, you'll discover that the lighter, freer, more abundant life you've always wanted has been waiting for you all along—"buried under everything you own."[11]

Inner Decluttering Tool: Consider the Lighter Way

In Matthew 11:28–30, Jesus reminds us that there is another way to live, a lighter way. But taking up the easy yoke of Jesus sometimes requires radically altering the trajectory of our lives.

Which areas of your life align with the easy yoke of Jesus? Which areas don't?

- your habits related to consumerism
- the speed at which you venture through life
- your practice of spending time in silence and solitude
- how you choose to spend the Sabbath

Don't judge your habits; just gather awareness. Minimalism is an invitation to find rest for your soul. Ask the Holy Spirit to help you align your choices with his lighter way.

Outer Decluttering Tool: Create a Mission Statement

Throughout history, many people—Jesus included—have used minimalism to support their life's mission. They didn't let go of superfluous possessions because material things are bad. They opted to live with less stuff because doing so freed them to do more of what mattered.

Companies and teams often develop a mission statement. Why? Increased alignment. When your mission becomes clear, your actions can better align with your purpose.

Write a one-sentence mission statement. Ask yourself this question:

If I were to die tomorrow, what would I most regret being unable to do?[12]

My answer: grow old with my husband and raise our kids into adulthood. My mission statement: I want to be present to my family, to really know and enjoy them, and to reflect God's love to them.

Maybe yours is a work-related goal or a humanitarian one. Whatever your answer is, minimalism will give you more space to live out your ambitions. A home with less stuff will free you to focus on your God-given mission— and lead you closer to a life of increased purpose and fulfillment.

Post your mission statement somewhere you will see it often.

3

REDEFINING RICH: A CLOSER LOOK AT MONEY

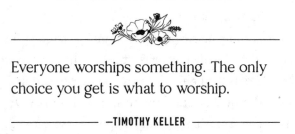

Everyone worships something. The only
choice you get is what to worship.

— TIMOTHY KELLER

We dwell in one of the wealthiest nations on the face of the earth. We have been raised in a cultural milieu that often places money on a pedestal.

Consider the following statistics:

- The average American has four credit cards in their wallet.[1]
- The average debt for indebted households is more than $16,000.[2]
- Each year in the US, more money is spent on shoes, jewelry, and watches than on higher education.[3]
- According to a recent YouGov survey, 70 percent of US

adults are indebted, including 78 percent of Gen Xers, 74 percent of baby boomers, 70 percent of millennials, and 44 percent of Gen Zers.[4]

- As of January 2023, 60 percent of US adults, including even four in ten high-income consumers, live paycheck to paycheck.[5]

Some of this debt is a result of factors outside of people's control—costly medical conditions, economic inflation, or an unexpected job loss. But some of it is self-inflicted, and that's where we have agency.

Money's allure coaxes many of us into pursuing things that, in the end, don't really matter. But here's the greater problem, one that Jesus is trying to warn us about: Attraction to material things diminishes our draw to spiritual things. Opting for love of money is opting for dulled spiritual sensitivity. When money captivates our mind and heart, we anesthetize ourselves to the Holy Spirit's movements, and eventually we lose our reliance on God.

Scripture talks a lot about money. The Bible includes roughly 2,350 verses about the topic, and in sixteen of his thirty-eight parables, Jesus used money to teach us spiritual truths.[6] The only subject Jesus taught about more is the kingdom of God.

Jesus's main takeaway? Love of God and love of money are incongruent, antithetical, clashing, incompatible. They don't coexist. In his Sermon on the Mount, Jesus said, "No one can serve two masters. Either you will hate the one and love the other, or you will be devoted to the one and despise the other. You cannot serve both God and money" (Matthew 6:24). Notice Jesus didn't say you "shouldn't" be devoted to both God and money. He says you "cannot" be. The two are polar opposites. You have to choose a side.

But in choosing to love God, do we have to completely disavow money? Are we to evade any money-related endeavor in the name of Jesus? The problem isn't money itself but rather devotion to it. First Timothy 6:10 tells us, "For the love of money is the root of all kinds of evil."

Ultimately, money is a matter of the heart, a matter of allegiance.

In *Mere Christianity*, C. S. Lewis writes,

> One of the dangers of having a lot of money is that you may be quite satisfied with the kinds of happiness money can give, and so fail to realize your need for God. If everything seems to come simply by signing checks, you may forget that you are at every moment totally dependent on God. . . . Often people who have all these natural kinds of goodness cannot be brought to recognize their need for Christ at all until one day, the natural goodness lets them down, and their self-satisfaction is shattered. In other words, it is hard for those who are rich in this sense to enter the kingdom.[7]

As Lewis suggests, we're designed to place God, not money, at the center of our devotion. When the two become interchanged, regardless of how much money we have, life feels anything but rich.

Selfless Living

Money can bolster our love for Jesus and others, but only when we handle it with a generous mindset. While I'm all about investing in self-care to best pour ourselves into others, adopting a mentality of selfless living prepares us for a life of increased meaning and happiness.

Consider the story of Sadio Mané, a Senegalese soccer star.[8] Mané, whose salary tops $10 million annually, attracted international attention because of his iPhone 11. Counter to what you'd expect for a multimillionaire, Mané's phone was outdated and cracked.

But the phone was still functional, so Mané didn't see any need for an upgrade.

When asked in an interview with TeleDakar why he chose to keep the dilapidated phone, he responded,

Why would I want 10 Ferraris, 20 diamond watches, and two jet planes? What would that do for the world? I starved, I worked in the fields, I played barefoot, and I didn't go to school. Now I can help people.

I prefer to build schools and give poor people food or clothing. I have built schools [and] a stadium; we provide clothes, shoes, and food for people in extreme poverty. I give 70 euros (approx. $78) per month to all people from a very poor Senegalese region in order to contribute to their family economy. I do not need to display luxury cars, luxury homes, trips, and even planes. I prefer that my people receive a little of what life has given me.[9]

Mané's story of rising from extreme poverty has shaped his relationship with money. Even in a Western, stuff-obsessed culture, his roots keep him grounded in a life with less. He chooses a humble and modest life because it allows him to solve world problems. From his excess, he gives others a chance at a better life.

No matter our backgrounds, the same can be true for us. Journeying through life with a generous attitude toward money allows us to embrace money as though it's actually God's money, not ours—because it is (Romans 11:36).

Scripture tells us that material detachment and generosity can lead to a richer life. Brain science, too, supports this idea. A University of Pittsburgh study performed brain scans on participants who chose to help others and those who chose to do something to benefit themselves. Those who opted to serve others showed increased activity in the brain's reward centers and decreased activity in areas related to elevated stress, blood pressure, and inflammation.[10]

Living in solidarity with others—recognizing others as our brothers and sisters in Christ and caring for them as such—is good for both humanity at large and our own health. But the opposite—worrying about money—is nothing short of detrimental. I know from experience.

Money Worries

A 2013 US survey of nearly three thousand people reported that 71 percent felt worried about money.[11] Seventy five percent of Americans reported making enough money to live within their means.[12] No doubt some or many of those people fell into the 71 percent who worried about money. Considering these numbers, we can safely conclude that, while poverty is real and heartbreaking, not all financial anxiety is caused by legitimate financial need. Could many of these money-induced worries stem from created needs?[13] Absolutely.

When we're baited to believe that happiness lies in the next purchase, and that newer and bigger means better, we worry about how to acquire more while also placating our consciences with lines like "It's not *that* much debt." Enter the escalated inner conflict.

In my own story, money spurred me to worry. I had $40,000 in credit card debt and another $60,000 in graduate school loans. I could see only two solutions to my finance-induced worry. One, make more money. Or two, spend less of it. Both came with a bevy of stumbling blocks.

One, I was staying at home full-time. Last I checked, the title "stay-at-home mom" didn't involve an inward cash flow. And two, my allegiance had always been to stuff and more stuff. That was exactly how I'd dug myself into the hole of unhealthy finances, money worries, and a dulled spiritual life. That wasn't a return on investment to be proud of or a lifestyle to recommend.

Minimalism was my springboard to examining my relationship with money and making healthy changes. Life with no consumer debt seemed like a pipe dream. But if other minimalists questioned their buying habits and halted their overconsumption, then I could too.

In *The Year of Less*, minimalist author Cait Flanders documents her twelve-month experiment of banning shopping for everything except consumables (groceries, toiletries, gas for her car). In changing her habits, Flanders was able to dig her way out of $30,000 of consumer debt, realizing that "when you want less, you consume less—and you also need less money."[14]

The need for less stuff begets the need for less money, freeing you to work fewer hours and maybe even live off one income, if desired. You accumulate less debt and save more money.

"You might get 85 years on this planet," writes Flanders. "Don't spend 65 years paying off a lifestyle you can't afford."[15]

Financial Freedom

Adopting a minimalist lifestyle and mindset not only frees you from worry. It also paves the way for financial freedom. Instead of viewing purchases in terms of dollar amounts, consider them in terms of hours of your life spent working. When we overspend, we're paying for superfluous things with valuable hours of our life. We have to work more to make more money to keep up with our consumption habits. And it's precisely these buying habits that take away our financial freedom.

In The Minimalists' documentary, Dave Ramsey said, "We're buying things we don't really need with money we don't really have to impress people we don't really like. We're giving up our freedom for some stuff that's going to be worth nothing in next year's garage sale."[16]

Minimalism has the power to change this cycle.

A 2023 study conducted by the *Journal of Retailing and Consumer Services* explored the effects of minimalist practices on consumer happiness and financial well-being. Researchers found that "adopting a minimalist lifestyle saves substantial money."[17] This aligned with earlier studies reporting that minimalism saves money. According to the researchers, "Reducing purchases saves money on items that add no life value. [Minimalist] consumers adopt a prudent and thoughtful stance toward consumption. They balance their spending according to budget limitations, which avoids overspending and debt burdens."[18]

Here are seven additional ways that minimalism can save you substantial money and enable financial freedom:

1. **DEVELOPING SELF-AWARENESS.** When you have less stuff in your home to clean and care for, you have more down-time. Margin makes space for prayer and introspection, which is needed for developing self-awareness and self-acceptance. When you *truly* get to know yourself, you learn what triggers you to shop and what causes you to fill your life with stuff, and then you realize that nothing you buy can augment your self-worth. This self-knowledge leads to much less mindless consumerism and frivolous spending.

2. **NOT RENTING A STORAGE UNIT.** The United States now has 2.3 billion square feet of self-storage space. (The Self Storage Association, a nonprofit trade group, notes that, with more than seven square feet for every man, woman, and child, it's now "physically possible that every American could stand—all at the same time—under the total canopy of self-storage roofing.")[19] Owning less means you won't have a monthly storage unit fee, or in the words of Jerry Seinfeld, you won't have to "pay rent to visit your incarcerated possessions."[20]

3. **THINKING OUTSIDE THE BOX.** Instead of buying something new, minimalists first see if something they already

own could serve the same purpose. They think outside the box before spending. Baby wipes can clean your TV, keyboard, and mouse just as well as pricey electronics cleaners. Coconut oil can remove makeup as well as any expensive product.[21] And chilled metal spoons can alleviate eye bags as well as costly creams. By using what you already have, you save money.

4. **NOT BUYING DUPLICATE ITEMS.** Why own seven pairs of jeans when you only love one of them? Why own five spatulas when one will do the trick? This "less is more" mindset counters consumerism.

5. **BUYING MULTIUSE ITEMS.** Minimalists look to buy items that can serve them in multiple ways. Mason jars, for example, can be used as vases, food storage containers, and drinking glasses. Owning one item to serve multiple purposes saves money.

6. **OWNING A SMALLER HOME.** Minimalist living may inspire you to downsize. When you live in a smaller space, you have a smaller mortgage and spend less on utilities and home maintenance costs in general.

7. **SHOPPING INTENTIONALLY.** Minimalist living gives you the space and time to align your life with your values. When you do need to purchase something, you do it intentionally, making a purchase that supports the life you're creating. You no longer feel the need to shop just for fun or to buy something just because it's on sale.

When we stop throwing more and more money toward stuff, we untether ourselves from our debt, regain focus on what matters most, and increase our ability to pursue it.

Releasing Guilt around Money

Even when we regain some degree of financial health and renounce our love of money, we can still feel guilty spending it, especially if we are in debt. That guilt is usually anchored in internal money narratives that took root in childhood.

If you grew up hearing "We can't afford that" on repeat, it's likely you still feel bad buying certain items, regardless of how much money is in your bank account.

Ramit Sethi, author of *I Will Teach You to Be Rich*, said, "We have a very unhealthy relationship with money in this country. On one hand, we have a puritanical strain that tells us, do not buy anything and you're a bad person for having debt. On the other hand, we look on Instagram and see our friend is going to be in Bora Bora on Tuesday, so we book a trip even though we don't know how much we have in the bank. What paradoxical beliefs! Usually it's the consumerist one that wins, but we still feel guilty."[22]

Minimalist living has the power to redefine—and even heal—your relationship with money. When you begin realizing what matters, what constitutes your rich life, you gain guidance on where to spend money. According to Sethi, this can be the impetus needed to dig your way out of debt.

"A rich life is when you look at your life and go, wow, this feels amazing," Sethi said in a podcast. "You can have a rich life and still be in debt. You can have a rich life and not yet be where you want to be ultimately. The key is that your rich life is yours—not your parents', not your friends', but yours."[23]

Defining a rich life, even while wallowing in debt, helps

you attach positive emotions to money again. The first step? Dreaming big. Sethi suggests sitting down with your spouse (or by yourself, if single) and creating a ten-year bucket list. Spend some time praying over the list. Then choose one thing from the list that would make the next ten years amazing and rich. Be specific. If you want to learn Spanish, do you want to do that online or in a Mexico City immersion program? If you want to help orphans, do you want to donate to your church or go on their next mission trip to an orphanage in Honduras? Say you choose the trip. Decide the month you'll go, visualize your seat on the airplane, imagine what you'll be wearing—be specific. Then approximate what it will cost (how much do you need to save per year?). Set up a monthly automatic transfer from your checking account to your savings account. Each month you'll see you're getting closer to your goal, and each month you'll experience joy.

"What you're doing is you're recalibrating the way you talk about money," Sethi says. "It's dreamy and fun."[24]

When our consumer debt hit $40,000, digging our way out felt like an insurmountable task. I stared at the debt, felt disempowered, and then made choices that were disempowering, like compulsive spending to temporarily numb the guilt. I thought being in debt meant I couldn't spend at all, so I felt bad anytime I did, which only led to more spending to cover the bad feelings. Minimalism taught me how to be intentional about spending. I realized I couldn't have it all, but I also realized I didn't need it all.

This financial shift is possible for you too. Sethi suggests spending unapologetically on what you love as long as you cut costs mercilessly on what you don't love.

Fill in these blanks: I spend extravagantly on _____ and I cut costs mercilessly on _____.

Maybe you spend extravagantly on tipping and cut costs mercilessly on your house. Or maybe you spend extravagantly on experiences and cut costs mercilessly on your car. Maybe you spend extravagantly on causes you're passionate about and cut costs mercilessly on your clothing.

Minimalism taught me that if I wanted to live my rich life, I also had to be able to say, *This is not part of my rich life.*

Taking Control of Your Money

Although it might seem counterintuitive, Sethi does *not* suggest creating a monthly budget. Instead, he recommends compiling a "conscious spending plan."

---

4 Key Numbers in the Conscious Spending Plan (CSP)

1. Fixed costs, including rent or mortgage, utilities, car payments, gas, groceries, and especially debt payments. These should be 50–60% of your take-home pay.
2. Savings (emergency fund, money you don't need for a while). This should be 5–10% of your take-home pay.
3. Investments. These should be at least 5–10% of your take-home pay.
4. Guilt-free spending (whatever you've decided you spend extravagantly on). This should be 20–35% of your take-home pay.

Sethi says, "Know the four numbers and you will suddenly feel totally in control [of your finances]."[25]

Knowing these four numbers and owning them was how I broke my cycle of conspicuous spending and how we finally became debt free. I taped the numbers from our CSP inside our kitchen cabinet next to a line graph of our debt (so I could track the number monthly as it decreased). I began buying groceries with a sense of relief instead of remorse and could even treat myself, my kids, and our elderly neighbor with guilt-free ice cream cones at a nearby shop. Once I knew the groceries, the ice cream, and even extra tipping didn't rob us of our ability to be out of debt someday, I could spend money on them without agonizing over the purchase. And when my spending no longer triggered guilt, I didn't have negative emotions to bury with another purchase.

Creating a CSP is also how I shifted my inner narratives about money. My self-talk around money went from distorted ("I'm not good with money. I'm never going to get out of this debt. I'm just an overspender.") to positive and truth-based ("I'm great with money. We will get out of debt. I'm in control of my spending.").

As you move toward financial accountability, question your beliefs around money and resolve to learn about money regardless of your state in life. (Sethi's book is a great place to start.) Minimalism will save you money and encourage spending habits that can lead to debt-free living. But even if you're debt free, you won't be truly "free" until your relationship to money is healed.

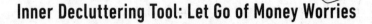

Inner Decluttering Tool: Let Go of Money Worries

C. S. Lewis said, "All these toys were never intended to possess my heart. My true good is in another world, and my only real treasure is Christ."[26] And Jesus said, "Where your treasure is, there your heart will be also" (Matthew 6:21).

Consider the following questions:

- Which has a greater claim on your heart, God or money? (Which do you think about more?)
- What feelings do you have at the thought of giving money away?

The next time you catch yourself worrying about money, stop and pray about how you can give some of it away. Then follow through on that plan. Here are some ideas:

- Tip a dollar extra.
- Buy coffee for the person behind you in line.
- Donate to a cause you're passionate about.
- Bring a meal to a friend in need or send them a DoorDash gift card.

Even small shifts toward generosity bless others and go a long way toward loosening your grip on money.

Outer Decluttering Tool: Create Your Conscious Spending Plan (CSP)

Revisit the conscious spending plan (CSP) mentioned earlier in this chapter and create your own.

- List your monthly fixed costs, savings, investments, and guilt-free spending. Post this information somewhere you can see it.
- Revisit your CSP once a month to adjust for changes.
- Pray about what God is calling you to spend freely on. Is there a cause or charity you feel called to support?

Taking control of your finances has the power to minimize your debt and increase your generosity.

CHAPTER

4

LETTING GO

Any half-awake materialist well knows—
that which you hold holds you.

—TOM ROBBINS

As I journeyed toward minimalism, I knew rationally that my stuff wasn't what mattered most. But I wasn't yet detached from my stuff emotionally. I'd invested in accumulating my possessions. I'd earned the money to pay for them and devoted the time to search for them (and, let's be honest, I'd found some amazing deals).

I had to remind myself over and over that a possession is like a bubble, or a dandelion blown in the wind, or a fireworks show. You observe it, enjoy it, and let it go. The things I owned were good, but they weren't the ultimate good, and I wasn't meant to cling to them as though they were.

I'd seen account after account of people from the Bible where Jesus asked them to give up their possessions to follow him: the rich young man (Matthew 19:21) and the apostles

Simon Peter, Andrew, James, and John (Mark 1:16–20). Postbiblical accounts showed the same: Saint Francis of Assisi, Saint Anthony of Egypt, Mother Teresa, not to mention their thousands of followers.

To others, Jesus had simply said, "Follow me," not "Divest yourself of everything you have and then follow me." Take Lydia of Thyatira, for example. Lydia ran an export business dealing in purple-dyed cloths (Acts 16:14). Purple goods were costly, so Scripture implies that Lydia was wealthy. She likely had a good-sized home and a good number of possessions. She encountered Paul on the Sabbath while gathering with other women at a nearby river. The Lord opened her heart to Paul's words, and she became a believer.

After her entire household accepted Christ as Savior and was baptized, Lydia invited Paul and Silas to stay in her home (Acts 16:15). Lydia again opened her home to Paul and Silas after their release from a Philippian prison, and her house became the meeting place of the first European church (Acts 16:40). Once a Christian, Lydia didn't jettison a single possession, but she did renounce her ownership of them. What had been hers before her conversion—home, business, and possessions—now belonged to the Lord.

In Scripture, there is no blanket statement that says every single follower of Jesus has to give everything away. But every follower of Jesus *is* called to give him everything.

Surrendering ownership of stuff wasn't an easy part of my journey—it felt contrary to my nature. Minimalism, I realized, would require a mindset shift. Before I pitched a single possession—outer or inner—God wanted me to give it all to him. God wanted access to everything: my stuff, my bank account, my relationships, my calendar, my thought patterns. He was and always had been their source, but I'd been white-knuckling them. I had wrapped my fingers around what was "mine" with a grip of steel. But clenched fists aren't conducive to letting go.

Loosening my grip meant turning over not only my hands, palms open to God, but also my ownership of any possession previously deemed mine. It was all his. I was simply the steward, which gave the term "stuff manager" a much different feel.

As I considered letting go, the question wasn't, "How do I give everything away?" but rather "How do I follow Jesus with everything?" Jesus was showing me that to follow him, for me, would mean to live with much less. That would require detaching from my things and also giving him access to everything—what I would declutter *and* what I would keep. If I wanted to build an inner home foundation cemented in Christ, I had to renounce my ownership before rolling up my sleeves and pitching my possessions.

Living with the End in Mind

A powerful personal experience finally made my detachment concrete. One December evening, while sitting in my car outside my favorite coffee shop—the one nestled on the corner of our town square, facade adorned with white globe lights—I had an overwhelming urge to call my grandma. (This was my paternal grandma, not my maternal one mentioned in the introduction.) I was new to these intuition-filled calls to action, but I was noticing them more now that I was focused less on stuff and more on God.

Eager to unload my daughters, sink into my favorite booth, and wrap my hands around a large, café-au-lait-filled mug, I tried to shake the feeling. My fingers grazed the car door's handle, but the voice telling me to call Grandma became deafening, so I grabbed the phone and dialed.

The conversation, as always, was soul-filling. I asked her questions about how in the world she managed raising nine kids. She shared a parenting tip, or at least some general encouragement, which I always welcomed. I promised to visit her in the not-too-distant future. She smiled—I could hear it in her voice—and said, "Oh, wouldn't that be nice. But a phone call is wonderful too."

After I had talked for twenty minutes, restless voices from the back seat cued the conversation's end. Eva requested a turn to talk, and in true five-year-old fashion, she excitedly spoke of the present moment and her long-awaited hot chocolate. Grandma said the call had meant so much and thanked me for it. I told her I loved her. And I told her goodbye.

Five days later, Grandma passed away unexpectedly. Nothing could have prepared us for the timing of her passing, and nothing could have left me more grateful for the evening when I postponed coffee to make that call.

As I placed a long-stemmed red rose on her casket one snowy December day, I was reminded again of the brevity of our time here on earth. I watched my warm breath form a white cloud as I exhaled into the frigid cemetery air. Then I watched it vanish.

Our journey through life is like that—transitory, fleeting, temporary. There is power in this perspective. Remembering death, living with the end in mind, propels us to use the time we have on earth to be less focused on inner and outer clutter and more focused on what truly matters.

The bottom line is this: You can't take your stuff with you. And chances are, when you come to the end of your life, you're not going to wish you had more of it. Moments of connection, beauty, and generosity are the "things" worth collecting as we journey through life.

Saint Francis of Assisi said, "When you leave this earth, you can take with you nothing that you have received—only what you have given." Love is what we've given, and love is what remains (1 Corinthians 13:13).

Keeping our own mortality in mind naturally shifts our focus away from our stuff. It increases our detachment and our propensity to let go.

In her book *Slow: Simple Living for a Frantic World*, Brooke McAlary explains how a simple writing prompt changed her life.[1] The prompt? Write your own three-sentence eulogy. The result? Amazing clarity on what truly matters in life.

In her eulogy, McAlary describes herself as a quick-to-laugh, creative, loyal, spontaneous person; a firm believer that we're all responsible to leave the world a better place than we found it; and a mom who raised daughters with both "roots and wings."

"I looked at my kids and husband and tried to imagine no longer being with them," McAlary writes. "The thought was painful, and I felt guilty. But what I also realized as I struggled to get the words on paper is that a eulogy doesn't leave any room for the unimportant things. The stuff we own, social media statistics, work success, having a nice home—I discovered that none of it really mattered."[2]

"The truth is none of us has any idea what the future holds," she continues. "I (now) knew what the most important, eulogy-worthy parts of my life were—family, adventure, having a positive impact in the world—I realized I wasn't living that life."[3]

While I wasn't scared of death, I was scared of leaving too much of my life unlived. I was terrified of having a legacy of tedious existence—being known for doing, amassing, and striving, but never really living. I feared living a life incongruent with what I'd want in my eulogy, which, I decided, included faith, family, presence, and adventure. I wanted to be remembered for beach trips where I ran through the waves barefoot and bedtime stories that ended in tears of laughter, for lingering on summer nights to gaze at stars and being present to the people I was blessed to be doing life with.

After that December, my view of possessions finally shifted.

Yours can too. The things to hold close, to be remembered for, aren't things at all.

Fixing your eyes on Christ (Hebrews 12:2) and thinking of things above (Colossians 3:2) creates space to declutter your soul and align your life with your desired legacy.

Observe each possession, enjoy it, then let it go. Because none of it is ever really ours in the first place.

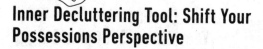

Inner Decluttering Tool: Shift Your Possessions Perspective

How do you view possessions? As permanent, defining pieces of your life, or as ephemeral objects? While the things of the world may be good and beautiful, the truly good, the truly beautiful, belong to a higher world. We can sense goodness and beauty in worldly things, but none of them last.

Which of the transient objects listed below can you most relate your possessions to?

- fireworks
- dandelions
- bubbles
- ocean waves

Take time today to pray with this visual in mind, and remind yourself that possessions are passing. Consider praying Paul's words in 1 Timothy 6:7—"We brought nothing into the world, and we can take nothing out of it"—to remind you that possessions are to be enjoyed in the moment but then released into God's hands.

Outer Decluttering Tool: Write Your Three-Sentence Eulogy

An anonymous quote I love reads, "No one is going to stand up at your funeral and say, 'She had a really expensive couch and great shoes.' Don't make life about stuff."

If you were to write your own three-sentence eulogy, would your possessions be included? Take time today to write it out and see. What is it that you want to be remembered for? Here are some possibilities:

- your personality
- your presence
- your faith
- your sense of adventure

A eulogy only leaves room for what's most important. Center your life on these "things," not your stuff.

5

AWAKENING TO THE SPIRIT WITHIN

Where the Spirit of the Lord is, there is freedom.

—THE APOSTLE PAUL (2 CORINTHIANS 3:17)

I've always opted for a deep, drawn-out conversation over snippets of small talk. In college I had a reputation for asking questions that some viewed as invasive and probing. But those were the questions that mattered. I didn't care much about someone's weekend plans; I wanted to know about the state of their soul.

And since this book is ultimately about you, if we were to go out for coffee, sit down, talk about your story, and discuss simplicity, that's likely where I would start.

"Your soul is not just something that lives on after your body dies," author Dallas Willard said. "It's the most important thing about you. It's your life."[1]

How *is* your soul?

I'm not looking for a conventional "good, bad, okay" response. I want to know if your soul is awake. Do you have moments when you feel your soul expand? Or is it static, listless, unresponsive? Is your soul awake? Is it in tune with the Holy Spirit?

An awake soul senses his inner promptings. A nudge here, a gentle jab there. It's the sudden urge to pray for a friend who's due with her fifth baby soon, only to find, after sending an encouraging text, that she's in early labor. It's the overwhelming tug to go check on my daughter and then finding her crying alone on the back porch. It's the impulse to call my grandma just days before her unexpected death.

An awake soul also senses the Spirit's outer movements. Simplicity makes space for us to absorb the subtleties in life and sense his handiwork. A zinnia sprout pushing through the earth, leaves bifurcating, opening toward the sun. An airplane's fluorescent jet stream searing through pink-orange clouds at sunset. A grandchild racing toward open arms with expectant eyes.

The Holy Spirit fills those moments, and when in tune, our soul expands.

"Every time you have experienced truth, goodness, or beauty, you have met the Holy Spirit," says pastor Edward Ahn. "Anytime you have encountered the beauty of God's creation, or the lovely face of a person, or the goodness of someone's love, or any truth that has captivated your heart and nourished your soul, you have met the Holy Spirit in such instances."[2]

Encountering the Holy Spirit and then handing him the

reins is of utmost importance. When God writes the story of your life and my life, it's going to be much greater than whatever manuscript we're attempting to self-publish (the small plans we have for our lives). A life well-led is a life that's God-led.

If we miss out on this union with the Holy Spirit, we end up "misliving," as philosopher William Irvine calls it. In his book *A Guide to the Good Life*, he writes,

> There is a danger that you will mislive—that despite all your activity, despite all the pleasant diversions you might have enjoyed while alive, you will end up living a bad life. There is, in other words, a danger that when you are on your deathbed, you will look back and realize that you wasted your one chance at living. Instead of spending your life pursuing something genuinely valuable, you squandered it because you allowed yourself to be distracted by the various baubles life has to offer.[3]

Are you in tune?

Distracted?

God wants to be our moment-to-moment companion. He wants to enter our inner homes and guide us toward plans greater than we can imagine. His guidance is available to us, but it's up to us to make space in our souls for him to act.

Jesus himself urged his followers to consider the importance of their soul in relation to the things of this world. In Matthew 16:26, Jesus asks, "What good will it be for someone to gain the whole world, yet forfeit their soul?" To forfeit means to lose or surrender. Has your soul been lost, numbed, inadvertently overtaken by the clutter of this world? Have you hung the white flag of surrender over the front door of your inner home?

Behind the Door of the Soul

Awakening to the Holy Spirit requires a greater understanding of the correlation between our outer and inner homes. An outer home, by its nature, is meant to be a foreshadowing of heaven. Home is where he longs to call us after our earthly journey is done.

Heaven is the eternal home he's created. And this desire for heaven—for home—is written in every human heart. It's no wonder we crave home. Author Jen Pollock Michel said, "In the beginning of time, God made a home for his people (a garden) and at the end of time God will make a home for us (a city)."[4] The original homemaker is God. And we, made in his image, are designed with a desire to create a home.

While God gave us the desire to create an outer home, he also created an inner home within every human being. Consider Paul's words to the Corinthians: "Do you not know that your bodies are temples of the Holy Spirit, who is in you, whom you have received from God?" (1 Corinthians 6:19). Our soul is not meant to be just a home for the Holy Spirit, but a temple.

Saint Teresa of Ávila explored this idea of an inner home in her work *The Interior Castle*. She wrote, "I thought of the soul as resembling a castle, formed of a single diamond or very transparent crystal, and containing many rooms, just as in Heaven there are many mansions."[5] She suggested that "the door by which we must enter this castle is prayer." God waits for us there. Yet he gives us the freedom to choose how much space we allow for him in our soul.

Do you have space for God's presence within you?

In *Theology of Home*, Carrie Gress writes, "Our homes can readily reveal what is happening behind the door of our soul."[6] Your external environment can serve as a lens to your inner environment.

Take a close look at the state of your outer home. Not in a judgmental, "shoulding" way, but with an open, curious spirit. Look around, pause, and ask yourself honestly, "What is my home reflecting back to me?" Does it reflect chaos and distraction? Does it reflect peace and calm? Are those accurate descriptors of your inner home as well?

There's a story of a beggar who, on his deathbed, gives his son the tools of his trade: a derelict cloth bag and a dirty bronze bowl. The son graciously receives his father's begging tools and begins using them. One day, a gold merchant approaches and drops a coin into the bronze bowl. The gold merchant, upon hearing the sound that the coin made, asks, "Can I see your bowl?" He examines the bowl and turns excitedly to the befuddled beggar.

"Why are you begging?" the merchant exclaims. "You're a rich man! This bowl is made of *gold*."

As Christians, we often don't see the treasure we have in the outpouring of the Holy Spirit. Jesus told his disciples that the Father would send the "Spirit of truth," who "lives with you and will be in you" (John 14:16–17). And so it is with us. Our very souls become the dwelling place of God. To paraphrase Augustine, the Lord is closer to us than we are to ourselves.

Though we may read and accept this fundamental truth,

our daily attunement to divine intimacy is continually in flux. How do we steady and deepen our connection with God's presence within us? We make space for our souls to wake up (Psalm 57:8). An uncluttered soul is an awake soul—a soul deeply aware that the very Spirit and life of God dwell within our inner home.

Soul-Filling Work

All this talk about making space for the Holy Spirit prompts another question: What do I want the inner rooms of my soul to be filled with? Minimalism isn't so much about what you want to let go of but what you want to keep. The same idea applies to the inner home. What do we want to keep, to materialize, in our souls?

Paul, in his letter to the Galatians (5:16–25 ESV), enumerates what fills Spirit-led souls:

> But I say, walk by the Spirit, and you will not gratify the desires of the flesh. For the desires of the flesh are against the Spirit, and the desires of the Spirit are against the flesh, for these are opposed to each other, to keep you from doing the things you want to do. But if you are led by the Spirit, you are not under the law. Now the works of the flesh are evident: sexual immorality, impurity, sensuality, idolatry, sorcery, enmity, strife, jealousy, fits of anger, rivalries, dissensions, divisions, envy, drunkenness, orgies, and things like these. I warn you, as I warned you before, that those who do such things will not inherit the kingdom of God.

But the fruit of the Spirit is love, joy, peace, patience, kindness, goodness, faithfulness, gentleness, self-control; against such things there is no law. And those who belong to Christ Jesus have crucified the flesh with its passions and desires. If we live by the Spirit, let us also keep in step with the Spirit.

The first list is composed of things that separate us from Jesus. Again, while there is nothing inherently bad about the flesh, the material, or the worldly, holding them as the highest good enslaves us. "When I hold on to the wrong things, the wrong things hold on to me,"writes Emily P. Freeman in the article "A Soul Minimalist's Guide to Letting Go."[7] These "wrong things" need to be jettisoned to live a free, Spirit-filled life.

The second list includes the fruit of a life lived in God. Love, joy, peace, patience, kindness, goodness, faithfulness, gentleness, and self-control can overtake your inner home when it serves as a sanctuary for the Holy Spirit—a clutter-free space where he can move freely.

It's not hard, tedious work for an orange tree to produce oranges. There's zero drudgery involved. It happens naturally. The tree blossoms, then several months later, oranges grow. The same is true for us if we welcome the Holy Spirit into our lives.

With more space and depth to our souls, with less clutter and chaos in our lives, the Holy Spirit can infuse us with more of his life-giving power. And it's that power that fully awakens our souls, pulls us in step with Jesus, produces fruit, and leads us to live lives that matter.

Having an uncluttered inner home doesn't mean evading hardship or suffering. But it does promise a place of inner peace—an inner meeting place with Jesus—that becomes your source of strength. A place you can return to anytime because he waits there for you.

Inner Decluttering Tool: Tune In to "Holy Spirit Moments"

Begin your day by tuning in to the presence of God's Spirit within you.

- Pray Psalm 57:8: "Awake, my soul!"
- Ask the Holy Spirit to come and fill your heart and occupy every space within your inner home.
- Worship with the song "Holy Spirit" by Jesus Culture or "Fall Afresh" by Jeremy Riddle.

Now look for "Holy Spirit moments" throughout your day when you feel him move within or when you experience truth, goodness, or beauty without. Begin a journal and record two to three "Holy Spirit moments" daily.

Outer Decluttering Tool: Create Beauty in Your Home

Anytime you have encountered beauty, you've encountered the Holy Spirit. Make a space in your home more beautiful today.

This may look like one of the following:

- placing fresh flowers on your kitchen table
- decluttering a kitchen countertop and keeping it clear
- filling a bowl with brightly colored fruits or veggies and displaying it in the kitchen
- making your bed
- lighting a candle
- displaying artwork or a photo you love

Whenever you see this beautiful space or thing, let it serve as a reminder that the Holy Spirit dwells within you. And when your mind drifts to him, ask him for an outpouring of his peace and guidance in your life.

CHAPTER

6

INNER DECLUTTERING
CHALLENGES

Whether you think you can or think you
can't — you're right.

—HENRY FORD

I woke up before the sun on a winter Saturday. Pink hues
lingered in the eastern sky, foretelling a breakthrough—
where was mine? My grandma's passing to her heavenly home
just two weeks prior had spurred me into let-it-go mode. I'd
been removing knickknacks here, broken toys there, but I
had hardly made a dent. My home environment still enabled
entropy. I still wallowed in overwhelm.

I stood, coffee in one hand, empty trash bag in the other,
eyeing the junk drawer nestled in the kitchen corner. After a
few determined tugs, the drawer budged, spilling a large pile
of papers and sticky notes onto the dark green linoleum.

I felt a familiar surge of anger. Then guilt. My decluttering efforts were mess-inducing. They felt futile. Stepping away from the paper-covered corner, I slouched onto a kitchen chair. I pushed more paper piles away with one hand and nearly slammed my coffee mug down. Hot liquid splattered. I inhaled sharply.

Lord, give me patience.

Patience. The fourth fruit of the Spirit Paul lists in Galatians. But I didn't feel patient; rather, I felt like grabbing my phone, scrolling Amazon, and purchasing something.

Chasing another purchasing-based high could deaden anger, but it could also deaden the Holy Spirit's movements within my soul. Purchasing and amassing possessions may suppress hard feelings temporarily, but it turns out that numbing the bad also numbs the good. To move through the tough emotions holding you back, you have to *feel* them.

I scanned the kitchen table. A preschool welcome letter, now partially covered in coffee splotches, lay within reach. Grabbing a pen from under an adjacent paper pile, I scribbled across the blank back of the paper. I recorded every angry thought and then countered it with truth:

- My home environment is out of control. *I am working to build a home environment that will support me.*
- My home environment is dirty. *Owning less will mean an easier-to-clean home.*
- I feel like nothing more than a full-time stuff manager. *My life will be fulfilling with less stuff.*
- I can't be present to loved ones, even God, because I'm surrounded by soul-numbing clutter. *Less stuff will free me to focus on who matters.*

I reread my words, which had given my emotions space to speak. I then ripped them into confetti-like shreds. Hedging my bets that the welcome letter contained no pressing preschool information, I stood and sprinkled its remains in the trash. Immediately I felt lighter.

Cue an aha moment—an epiphany that outer change would be fueled by having tools to ground my thoughts in truth, not anger or guilt.

This didn't mean anger and guilt were gone forever. But a layer of guilt and anger that had rendered me paralyzed, unable to dive in and fully let go of my possessions, had been removed with truth.

I could breathe more deeply now. I felt *ruah*—which in Hebrew can mean "breath" of the Spirit—filling previously occupied places in my soul, as if I was receiving more patience with each deep inhale. I felt more alive, more serene, more ready to persevere.

Half Method, Half Mental

As I discovered that Saturday morning, your most formidable decluttering barrier is often yourself. We all have distorted beliefs that, if left untouched, block us from reaching our goals. Some stem from childhood, while others are simply a product of how our brains function.

Author and life coach Shira Gill writes in her book *Minimalista*, "As soon as you set a big goal, your brain will almost inevitably start to have a tantrum. It will tell you your goal is too hard or complicated or that you will fail. Your brain is just doing its job. It wants to keep you safe, and anything new will feel like danger to the primitive part of your brain."[1]

For most people, the challenge is often twofold: one, overcome a change-resistant brain, and two, uproot inner narratives that aren't grounded in truth.

The apostle Paul writes to the Philippians, "Finally, brothers and sisters, whatever is true, whatever is noble, whatever is right, whatever is pure, whatever is lovely, whatever is admirable—if anything is excellent or praiseworthy—think about such things" (4:8).

God wants our minds to meditate on truth. Our thoughts shape our actions, rendering them in or out of alignment with God's purposes and plans for our lives. If thoughts spur our actions, then decluttering is half method and half mental.

Joyce Meyer, author of *Battlefield of the Mind*, writes, "You cannot have a positive life and a negative mind."[2] I would echo her by saying, "You cannot have an uncluttered home and a negative mind."

Dr. Daniel Amen suggests that automatic negative thoughts—what he calls ANTs—can be eliminated by watching your thoughts closely.[3] Once an ANT is identified, it must be smashed by a truth statement. Amen has labeled nine types of ANTs, including the following:

1. "Guilt Beating" ANTs (anytime the word *should* is used: *I should have a more decluttered home by now.*)
2. "Always or Never Thinking" ANTs (anytime the word *always* or *never* is used: *I'll never have time to declutter my home.*)

3. "Labeling" ANTs (anytime you attach a negative label to yourself or someone else: *I am such a mess, just like my home.*)
4. "Fortune Telling" ANTs (anytime you predict the worst possible outcome: *My house is overrun by stuff. It's too big of a job to declutter it.*)
5. "Blaming" ANTs (anytime you blame something or someone else for the problems in your life: *It's my kids' fault that my home is cluttered.*)

Every thought pattern we entertain changes our brain chemistry for better or worse. (Think: more negative thoughts, less dopamine, and more desire to go buy something to drum up more dopamine.) A negative self-talk spiral that drains dopamine lays the groundwork for retail therapy and impulse shopping. Rooting our self-talk in truth not only can help us persevere on our simplicity journey but also can break our need to buy more.

If you're ready to declutter your physical home, it's time to channel your inner exterminator. Amen recommends writing down each negative thought and then a truth statement that counters it.

ANT: I should have a more decluttered home by now.
Truth: I'm committed to this process and will finish at just the right time.

Did you feel your brain shift gears as you read that? Each thought is a chemical reaction. Let's try another.

> **ANT:** I am such a mess, just like my home.
> **Truth:** I am God's beloved child. My home will soon
> support me.

Sense the difference? Let's do one more.

> **ANT:** I'll never have time to declutter my home.
> **Truth:** I find time for what's important to me. This is
> important to me.

Unless we develop the skill of catching automatic negative thoughts and smashing them with God's truth, they remain just that: automatic. Subconscious. Writhing below our level of awareness, wreaking havoc without our consent.

God has given us the crucial task of centering our thoughts on the true, noble, and lovely. Philippians 4:8 may emit a vibe of simplicity, as if "thinking on the good" is easy. It's not. To have constant awareness and control of your mind is a skill, not second nature, especially in today's world of social media and marketing. (Reminder: Subliminal messages are a science; marketers are trained to toy with your subconscious.)

Researchers at the University of Southern California Laboratory of Neuro Imaging found that humans have up to seventy thousand thoughts per day.[4] According to the National Science Foundation, 80 percent of our thoughts are negative and 95 percent of our thoughts are repetitive.[5]

Read that again. Think the Enemy taps into this? Absolutely. Lies—anti-truths—are his jam. But it's by Spirit and truth that we're transformed into the image of Jesus. The nebulous, the deceitful—they simply can't stay. Not if the author of our souls is going to take up residence on the inside. And not if we're going to do impediment-free decluttering work on the outside.

Catching and squashing the ANTs with truth statements is as important throughout the decluttering process as your decluttering method. It's arguably more important. If your subconscious berates you with "shoulds" as you clear out junk drawer contents—*I should be doing this faster* or *I never should have bought all this stuff*—then you'll likely quit halfway through the task. If you change your self-talk to be more truthful—*I'm doing the work needed to create a lighter, more meaningful life* or *I forgive myself for everything I bought and don't use*—you can remove the internal roadblocks. And a barrier-free path makes for a smoother journey.

Breaking Down Cognitive and Emotional Decluttering Barriers

For many of us, letting go of clutter is work. Now, there are some people, like Ryan Nicodemus of The Minimalists, who can host a packing party, box up every possession as though he were moving, unpack only the essentials over a two-week span, and then donate every unopened box. But for most of us, the minimalism plunge is a bit more protracted. We want to make deliberate decisions, hold almost every item we own, question the value it adds to our lives, and determine its fate.

Research reveals a number of cognitive and emotional barriers that can make it difficult for us to let go of our physical possessions.

In the cognitive realm, we face:

- **THE MERE EXPOSURE EFFECT.** The more we are exposed to something, the more it will become favorable to us. We become attracted to our possessions simply by being regularly exposed to them.[6] (*I see these books every day and feel like they belong here, so I'll keep them even though I don't particularly like them.*)
- **THE STATUS QUO BIAS.** Any decrease from the status quo is perceived as a loss, even when there are financial advantages to selling or changing things we possess.[7] (*I want to downsize my house, but I've always lived in one this size, so I probably won't change.*)
- **THE ENDOWMENT EFFECT.** We overvalue things we own simply because we have ownership. We place a higher value on an item we own than on an identical item we don't own.[8] (*I'm keeping this outfit because it's mine, even though I don't really need or use it.*)

In the emotional realm, we face:

- **GUILT.** We self-sabotage, making the cluttered state of our home a moral affair. We feel bad for discarding items we spent good money on. Or we feel like we should keep certain gifts we were given, even though we don't want or use them. (*I don't want all this china, but it was my grandmother's, so I should keep it.*)
- **FEAR.** We're afraid we'll need an item in the future, so we keep it even though we haven't needed it in years. Sometimes our memories of a person or event are linked to an item. We fear losing the memory, so we hold on to the item. (*I don't want all these souvenir magnets from*

when I traveled through Europe, but I'm afraid I'll lose the memories if I get rid of them.)

- **SELF-DOUBT.** We deploy 101 excuses for why we can't declutter our home because deep-down we don't truly believe we can. (*I can't really change my spending habits and keep my home clutter free.*)

Our human nature can make relinquishing possessions downright hard at times—even possessions that are unwanted and unloved. Many of us simply aren't naturally wired to let go of our stuff. But neither are we wired to be weighed down by trinkets and tchotchkes—enter the stress, anxiety, spiritual numbness. Thankfully, there are tools that can help us overcome these decluttering barriers.

1. **RECOGNIZE BIASES.** When faced with an item you're struggling to let go of, dig deep. Ask yourself questions to uncover any biases. Would you buy this item today? If yes, how much would you pay for it? Do you feel like you "should" keep it, or do you love or use it? Are you afraid you'll need it in the future or fear you'll lose a memory if you donate it? Are you worried about what someone would think if you let go of it? Addressing the real reasons you're hanging on to an item you don't really want will make it easier to let it go.

2. **GET CLEAR ON YOUR VALUES.** As noted previously, when you're clear on your values, letting go of your possessions becomes easier. Maybe, after God, your family is most important to you, but you feel unable to be present to them because of your cluttered home.

Understanding that less stuff means more quality time with loved ones can override any of your reasons for holding on to unwanted possessions.

3. **LOOSEN THE ATTACHMENT WITH TIME.** If you feel unable to let go of an item, store it away for a while. Remember we're more biased to keep things we see daily (per the "mere-exposure effect" mentioned earlier). After a couple of months, revisit the item. See if your attachment has loosened and you're now able to let it go.

4. **REALIZE MEMORIES STAY WHEN POSSESSIONS GO.** Physical possessions can trigger memories, but remember that your memories are stored in your mind, not in your stuff. And there are ways to continue enjoying those memories without the possessions. Take pictures of items before donating them. Or keep a minimal amount—say, one china teacup instead of all twelve. Realize that when you let go of an item, you're freeing up physical and mental space, allowing you to live more fully in the moment and make new memories.

5. **FORGET OTHER PEOPLE'S OPINIONS.** Avoid owning items simply to keep up with the Joneses. Status symbols aren't worth keeping. If you're holding on to something because it was a gift, remember the gift has already fulfilled its purpose of expressing love. You've said thank you, felt the love, and are now free to let it go if you don't need or like it.

6. **OVERCOME GUILT WITH GRATITUDE.** Decluttering guru Marie Kondo suggests using gratitude to help overcome guilt. She says that many people may feel guilty when letting go of items, but expressing gratitude (she recommends

verbally thanking the item for its service) will dramatically lessen the feeling of guilt.[9]

7. **TAP INTO TRUST.** If you're holding on to something simply because you're afraid you'll need it in the future, consider trusting that you will have what you need when you need it. Say, for example, you own fifteen cookbooks, really use only two, and keep the rest just in case you need a recipe from them sometime. Trust that you'll find a good recipe online instead, and let the unused books go.

"Just in Case" Thinking

A main reason we hold on to our possessions is "just in case" we need them in the future. This type of thinking is usually rooted in fear or a need for control. If you find yourself stuck in "just in case" thinking, here are three tips to try.

1. Fill in the Blank

Author Courtney Carver writes that one reason we hold on to things just in case is because we don't finish the sentence. Sure, it's easy to say we will keep something just in case. But just in case of what? Articulate what you think might happen. Say it out loud to yourself. Say it out loud in front of other people. The more you get your justification out in the open, the more reasoning you can apply to it.

You: "I need to keep seven inherited vases in my kitchen cabinet just in case . . . some of them break."

Also you: "Have I ever broken a vase? No. Okay, two will do."

2. Realize "Just in Case" Means Never

"Just in case means never," writes Carver.[10] The hard truth is that we rarely use or enjoy the stuff we keep just in case. Take a good look at your junk drawer, the boxes in your garage, or the back of your closet for proof.

You: "I need this entire box of sentimental items just in case I want to relive all these memories."

You (realizing that "just in case" means never): "I haven't opened the box in two years. I'll keep my three favorite pieces, display and enjoy them, and let go of the rest. If I want to, I can take a picture of the stuff I let go of to preserve the memory."

Carver says, "Admitting that 'just in case' means never allows us to stop procrastinating and invites us to let go and stop living in fear."[11] When we stop living in fear of not having enough, we stop holding on just in case.

3. Use the 20/20 Rule

The Minimalists' 20/20 Rule is a powerful way to let go of "just in case" items.[12] This rule suggests letting the possession go if . . .

- you can replace it for less than twenty dollars
- *and* you can replace it in less than twenty minutes.

Should I let go of that fuchsia lipstick I wore once to my brother's wedding? What about those multiple spatulas? Or those rarely used coffee mugs? Run the item through the 20/20 Rule and the answer is usually a unanimous yes.

In my experience, you rarely need to replace the things you decide to relinquish using this rule. You won't miss what you didn't actually need.

Overcoming our natural tendencies to hold on to our stuff takes a lot of work. The good news is that we don't have to do it alone. In Eugene Peterson's *The Message*, he paraphrases Ephesians 3:20–21 by writing, "God can do anything, you know—far more than you could ever imagine or guess or request in your wildest dreams! He does it not by pushing us around but by working within us, his Spirit deeply and gently within us."

Any project, home decluttering included, is a tandem gig. We do the work by God's grace and with the guidance of the Holy Spirit. Augustine said, "Without Him, we cannot. Without us, He will not."[13] We are cocreators of this life with God, and with his grace and the right tools, that life is about to become a whole lot simpler.

Inner Decluttering Tool: Ask for Spiritual Fruit

Ask God for help in breaking down cognitive and emotional barriers. A spiritual mentor once told me that the most important word in the Bible is *with*. God wants to be with us every step of our earthly journey, which includes our decluttering journey.

Consider asking for the following fruits:

- patience with yourself (e.g., if you feel angry with yourself for frivolous past purchases or the amount of clutter in your home)
- self-love (e.g., if you're feeling guilty about your clutter)
- gentleness (e.g., if you're having self-sabotaging thought patterns)
- self-control (e.g., if you're tempted to buy more stuff you don't need or tempted to entertain negative thoughts)

Ask him for the spiritual fruit you need. He's got you and always will.

Outer Decluttering Tool: Practice ANT Catching

Cognitive distortions simply do not serve us. Smash them by getting them out of your head and onto paper, where they can be countered with truth. Here's how:

- Designate a consistent window of time each day to observe, catch, and smash your automatic negative thoughts (ANTs). For example, choose 10:00–10:15 each morning while you're working in the kitchen.
- Place a paper and pencil on the countertop and write down each negative thought as it comes up. Don't judge it; just record it.
- Immediately write a truth statement next to the negative statement.
- Continue catching negative thoughts as they arise for the full fifteen minutes and repeat daily for ten days.
- After the ten days, tackle one decluttering task that previously felt too difficult to begin. With consistent, truthful self-talk, you will be able to complete the project.

Consider googling "Dr. Amen's 9 'species' of ANTs" to learn more about the nine types of automatic negative thoughts. Remember, each thought we have is a chemical reaction. As ANT catching becomes second nature, you are building a better brain and dismantling roadblocks that keep you from decluttering.

CHAPTER

7

OUTER DECLUTTERING CHALLENGES

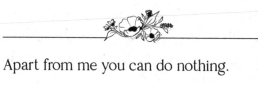

Apart from me you can do nothing.

—JESUS (JOHN 15:5)

Conquering the kitchen drawer felt good. Really good. It could open and close freely again, I now knew its contents, and everything was neatly ordered inside. But the high was short-lived. Any inkling of tranquility and order dissipated at the sound of small feet pattering on our wooden split-level stairs. Of course, I welcomed and embraced Eva's presence. But the exorbitant number of trinkets and random clothes she'd decided to haul downstairs along with her this particular morning? Not so much.

What motivated her to grab *everything* in sight and trail it around the house? And then it hit me. The environment was dictating her behavior. She was putting on a "stuff parade" simply because it was there.

In this moment, I recognized a major external decluttering roadblock: My decluttering method was all wrong.

I'd read to start small, in nonsentimental, contained spaces—a bathroom drawer, a kitchen pantry shelf, the junk drawer. The momentum from these small decluttering wins was supposed to carry me from an uncluttered bathroom drawer to an uncluttered bathroom to an entirely uncluttered home.

While starting in nonsentimental kitchen drawers worked well for some people, I wasn't one of those people. This plan didn't address my overwhelm. If anything, it increased my angst. I had just sacrificed an hour of much-needed sleep to declutter a drawer, only to turn around and continue managing randomly-strewn-about stuff. The kitchen drawer wasn't the biggest source of my stress. Sure, it was now nice to look at and delivered the "feel goods" of finishing a project. But what good were these sentiments if they vanished the minute I closed that drawer and returned to my everyday life?

Eva, hands full of sweater dresses, multiple blankets, a disheveled slinky, her toothbrush, and mismatched costume jewelry, entered the kitchen and unloaded her haul, forming a hefty pile beside the kitchen chair. I was torn between uttering a dejected "Nooo," barking strict orders, and simply being the observer. I chose the last one.

If my decluttering efforts were going to lighten life and restore function in our home, then I needed to tackle the clutter by category—starting with the one causing the most stress and then continuing through our home.

It was as though my daughter, in welcoming me with a pile of stuff, had inadvertently hand-delivered me the decluttering plan I was missing. Her stuff-laden arms led to my clarity. For life to be lighter, I had to focus on letting go of what was heaviest. What did it matter if I had an organized kitchen drawer when I was drowning in kids' clothes and toys? I needed to declutter in a way that felt less by the book and more aligned with my intuition, a way that would lead me to become rich in what mattered by releasing what was most keeping me from it.

You, too, can start decluttering your home in a way that allows you to make the biggest impact. Here are my recommendations:

1. Divide Your Clutter into Categories

Grab a pen and paper (or the notes app on your phone) and list out your clutter categories. Whatever comes to mind, write it out. There's no right or wrong way to do this. The following are some of my categories. Yours will likely look different, and they should—minimalism looks different for everyone.

Kids' clothes
My wardrobe
Kids' toys
Kitchen items
Paper
Kids' books
My books

Notice I didn't include "my husband's golf magazines" on my list. Focus on your own stuff and the stuff you're responsible to care for. (If your kids are young, then their stuff is your responsibility. See chapter 11 for tips on involving kids in the decluttering process.)

2. Assign a Brief "Why" for Each Category

Next to each clutter category, jot down a few words to remind yourself why you want to declutter this specific area. Here are some examples:

Kids' clothes
- ☐ Spend less time on laundry (and more time on the things that matter).
- ☐ Own an amount of clothes that our kids can fold and put away themselves.

Paper
- ☐ Spend less time looking for missing papers.
- ☐ Remove distracting (and stress-inducing) piles from the countertops.

3. Rate Each Category on a Stress Scale

Rate each clutter category on a scale of one to ten, ten being an extreme stress source and one being a minimal stress source. Go with your gut—no need to overthink it. Jot the number next to the category.

For me, kids' clothes were a ten. They flooded our home and were the bane of my existence. Kids' toys were a nine. I was constantly tripping over toy piles and stuffed animals that seemed to multiply overnight. Paper clutter was an eight. We had no system to manage our papers, and shuffling piles took up way too much of my time.

4. Tackle the Top-Rated Category First

The trick to decluttering with a bigger impact is tackling the top-rated clutter category first. Whatever area you rated a ten, start there. (If you have more than one area rated ten, flip a coin, draw straws—just choose one and start.) Decluttering your "tens" first ensures that each decluttering session will improve your daily life and your ability to function.

For me, the biggest clutter culprit was kids' clothes, so that's where I started. The results were life-changing, really. My kids started helping with laundry because the amount of clothes to manage was no longer overwhelming. I felt like I could breathe again in the laundry room and kids' room. And I created significant free time for myself. Remember, there is no right or wrong way to declutter. *You* determine the way that works best for you. You can chip away at your clutter, or you can knock it out in chunks. Either approach will create the space and breathing room you've been craving.

Finding Time to Declutter

Once you have your method down and you know the order of categories, another outer roadblock will likely arise: finding the time to declutter. You're about to journey into one of the most life-changing (or perhaps better said, life-reclaiming) projects you've ever undertaken. Be intentional about making time for it.

In my experience, decluttering your home is one of the best time investments you can make. The return on your investment is phenomenal. Invest a bit of time up front in decluttering your home, and soon you'll have fewer stuff-related to-dos, resulting in more free time in your daily life.

Studies show that decluttering reduces the amount of time spent on housework by 40 percent in the average home.[1] Let that stat sink in for a minute. That's almost half the number of housework-dedicated minutes of your life.

If you spend ten hours a week cleaning, organizing, and maintaining things, you could gain back four of those hours simply by having less stuff to manage. What would you do with four extra hours a week? (An extra sixteen hours a month; an extra 208 hours [8.5 days] a year.) Anything you've been wanting to do but haven't had the time! Connect with your kids, take up a new hobby, spend more time with friends, read books, exercise, cook—it's all waiting for you once your living environment contains less.

Here are seven ways to make time to declutter your home.

1. **REDUCE YOUR DISTRACTIONS.** If you're like most Americans, time spent scrolling social media and watching TV takes up several hours of your day. (On average, TV alone claims three hours.[2]) Each day, could you use one of those hours decluttering your home instead? I'm guessing so. You might miss your favorite reality show, but remember, time invested in decluttering now means much more time for other stuff later. Keep time spent on your phone to a minimum by deleting your social media apps for a while or by keeping your phone somewhere you can

hear it ring but not see it.

2. **SCHEDULE IT.** Find time to declutter your home by scheduling weekly or biweekly decluttering appointments with yourself, then show up for them—on time and ready to simplify. If you have children, hire a sitter or ask family or friends to help with childcare, just like you would for a real appointment. If you work full time, consider scheduling a fifteen-minute morning or afternoon decluttering work break. Or schedule a decluttering lunch where you either actually declutter or write out a decluttering plan for that day/week. Could you squeeze in some decluttering while listening to a training or meeting?

3. **GET UP EARLIER OR STAY UP LATER.** For those of you with small kids, finding time to declutter your home while they are sleeping is a great option. If you're a morning person, get up an hour early. If staying up late is more your thing, do that. Or do a bit of both. While I'm not one to overlook the importance of sleep, sacrificing a little here and there can go a long way toward decluttering your home.

If you set a timer and spend 15 minutes each morning (or evening) decluttering, that's 7.5 hours a month and 90 hours a year. Small, consistent efforts lead to big changes.

---

4. **THINK OUTSIDE THE BOX.** One of my favorite ways to find time to declutter during our initial purge was by playing hide-and-go-seek with our daughters. I'd put one donate bag and one trash bag on the kitchen table.

When it was my turn to seek, I'd take an extra-long time finding them and would slowly work my way through a kitchen cabinet or a closet during the game. I still like to play this game for maintenance decluttering (it's a great way to clear countertops during the day).

5. **DESIGNATE DECLUTTERING WEEKENDS.** Commit large chunks of your weekends (or whatever days you're off work) to decluttering your home. You could even use a day or two of vacation time and make it a long weekend. If you have small kids, you can declutter while your spouse spends quality time with them. Or if your kids are a bit older, you can involve them in the decluttering work. You can still mix in leisure time, like sorting through the contents of a junk drawer while listening to your favorite podcast.

6. **LET GO OF A COMMITMENT.** Temporarily withdraw from one of your regular commitments. Maybe pause your volunteering at your child's school, stop attending an optional meeting, or postpone a regular get-together with a friend. The fewer commitments you have for this season, the more time you'll have to declutter your home and minimize your possessions.

7. **WATCH FOR WINDOWS OF TIME DURING THE DAY.** Enter each day ready to watch for free moments that you can use to declutter your home. Maybe your kids are playing well together after breakfast. Tackle a drawer of clothes. Or maybe you have free time during their nap time. Go through a shelf in the hall closet. Keep decluttering at the top of your mind, and take action when the moment is right.

Decluttering is an investment in your relationship with your kids and others. Again, time spent decluttering today means more free time in the future, which you can spend fully engaged with those you love.

When Your Spouse or Family Isn't on Board

Studies suggest clutter can affect men and women differently. A 2010 study by Dr. Darby Saxbe found that in couples who live in cluttered spaces, women have higher cortisol levels during both the day and night (when levels normally drop).[3] Men also had elevated levels of cortisol *if* they did housework in the cluttered environment. Saxbe concluded, unsurprisingly, that the person most responsible for navigating the clutter tends to be the one most stressed out by it.

"Clutter is in the eye of the beholder," she said. "The people who talked about [the clutter] were the ones who had the cortisol response."[4]

So what can you do if you're the one talking about clutter but your loved ones aren't? What if you value a decluttered space but your loved ones don't seem to get it?

Here's the good news: Your loved ones don't have to be on board. It's that simple. You can still feel the spiritual and emotional benefits of decluttering by focusing on your own stuff. In the words of author Erica Layne, "You don't have to feel burdened by another person's reluctance to join in; you can choose to let go of your expectations and forge ahead on your own path."[5]

Control what you can control—*your* expectations and

actions, not those of others. However, it's normal to want your spouse to join in. So here are three things you can do to encourage them to try minimalism.

1. Delegate More Household Responsibilities

If you are primarily in charge of maintaining the home, your loved ones will become accustomed to that and begin to expect it of you.

Begin delegating small tasks to those around you. When loved ones realize how long a certain task takes (like picking up toys or doing dishes), they will likely be more open to owning fewer possessions in that area so as to cut down on work time.

Remember, the person who is responsible for navigating the clutter is the one who gets the most stressed about it. Let your loved ones do some clutter navigating so that they too feel the need for change.

2. Model the Benefits of Living with Less

As you focus on decluttering your own items, clear spaces will emerge around the home. You will begin to feel lighter, your mood will likely improve, and you'll have more free time on your hands. As your loved ones observe these changes, they will likely notice the benefits of living with less.

Neuroscience indicates that we often become like those we spend the most time with, thanks to mirror neurons in the brain. Our actions and improved emotional state can be contagious on a physiological level. In time, if we stay consistent with decluttering, our loved ones will likely begin imitating some of our actions and become more open to living with less.

3. Talk to Your Loved Ones about Clutter

Start the conversation about clutter and its effect on you. But be mindful about when and how you communicate. The best time to talk about clutter is not when it is making you feel super stressed. Instead, choose a time when you're calm and have your loved ones' full attention. Mention facts from an interesting study on clutter and well-being. (For example, you could say, "A study done at Princeton found that tidying your workspace can lead to more productivity."[6])

Observe your loved ones' response and give them the freedom to respond any way they choose. A few days later, make another emotionally neutral clutter-related comment. Maybe you mention how much more relaxed you feel in an orderly home. Or how much better you're sleeping now that the bedroom is decluttered. Keep the comments positive and consistent.

In the meantime, if your spouse is particularly messy and isn't yet on board with letting go of possessions, consider encouraging organization in subtle ways. If your spouse litters clothes across the closet floor, place a basket there and ask him to please place his clothes in it instead. If his keys and wallet are constantly on the kitchen counter, place an aesthetically pleasing storage container in the exact place this clutter routinely falls. A few simple systems can go a long way.

Still, it's likely that you'll sense some uncertainty or resistance from your spouse or your family. So tread lightly. Trust the process. And channel your energy toward decluttering your own stuff.

By now, the decluttering foundations have been laid. Return to chapters 6 and 7 anytime you approach a roadblock and need a decluttering boost. While the guidance in these chapters is helpful, you have the greatest Guide within. You've got this, not because of your decluttering prowess but because, ultimately, you're not conquering this project on your own.

Inner Decluttering Tool: Choose a Project Verse

Each New Year, it's common practice to choose a word for the year. It's a simple way to remind yourself of what's important and what you want to achieve, like having a personal motto or slogan.

Choose a Bible verse to ground your decluttering efforts. For example,

- I can do all this through him who gives me strength. (Philippians 4:13)
- Commit to the LORD whatever you do, and he will establish your plans. (Proverbs 16:3)
- The LORD is my shepherd; I shall not want. (Psalm 23:1 KJV)

Write your verse at the top of your Decluttering Plan (see the next tool) and entrust your house-clearing work to him.

Outer Decluttering Tool: Revisit Your Decluttering Plan

In her blog post "Dear Me, Lines to the Person I Want to Be," author Ann Voskamp writes, "Stress is a choice."[7] I would add, "Owning items that cause stress is a choice." Remember to see your clutter in stress-inducing categories. Revisit the decluttering plan that you started earlier in this chapter. Remind yourself which category (kitchen stuff, toys, etc.) prompts the most inner agitation.

Once you've identified this category, complete the following journal prompts:

- Why does this area cause you the most stress?
- Why do you want to declutter this area?

Knowing your "why" guides you as you continue your decluttering efforts.

Post your decluttering "game plan" somewhere you will see it daily, then follow it to efficiently create a clutter-free home.

PART 2

Decluttering the Main Floor / Heart

There is a God-shaped vacuum in the heart of each man which cannot be satisfied by any created thing but only by God the Creator, made known through Jesus Christ.

—ATTRIBUTED TO BLAISE PASCAL

CHAPTER

8

DECLUTTERING THE KITCHEN AND LETTING GO OF RESTLESSNESS

Calm, peace, and relaxation do not have
to do only with bodily or physical well-
being. They create a greater openness to
God, and at the same time they incarnate
God's peace within us, the peace that,
Paul writes, must "reign" in our hearts.

—WILFRID STINISSEN

Every morning during my journey toward minimalism, I
began my days in silence at the kitchen table—hands around
a hot drink, mind intermittently quiet, heart open to Jesus. I'd
invite him to take a seat and stay awhile. I told him I didn't really
know how to pray, but the peace that flooded my inner home
in these moments told me it didn't matter. We were together.

"You mustn't expect happiness from the things of the earth," wrote Gabrielle Bossis, "but solely from your way of communing with God."[1] During my quiet mornings, I was beginning to believe this truth. My heart's realigning and reopening was bringing me back to the heart of my Christian faith: Jesus.

The kitchen table, nestled in the heart of the home, was a visual reminder that my heart was being changed by an invisible reality. That table had adopted a new purpose, revitalized by the title "place of morning prayer." This idea of purpose, I realized, applied to the entire room. What was the purpose of this quaint, rectangular kitchen stretching from sink to basement stairs?

Although I had reclaimed the table as a place for morning devotion, the rest of the kitchen was still overrun with a lot of domestic flotsam—paper piles, forgotten Happy Meal toys, and expired pantry staples.

The physical chaos was a source of spiritual restlessness.

Being a catchall for randomness had left the room bereft of meaning, function, and purpose. Before deciding what to donate, trash, or keep, I needed clarity on the kitchen's role. So I started brainstorming on a paper scrap. "A clean, uncluttered, cozy place to gather," I wrote. "A place of peace, not chaos."

I would be spending a good deal of time here, and I wanted the feel of the room—once it was peaceful, not chaotic—to help me move through life at Mary's pace, not Martha's (Luke 10:38–42).

Just as the heart pumps blood to the body, the kitchen, the heart of the home, pumps ripples of serenity or chaos throughout the home. I wanted the kitchen to be a beautiful place that helped me raise my heart to God and be more present to those gathered around me.

But how?

The Power of Half

In *The Power of Half*, author Kevin Salwen documents his family's journey of letting go of half their possessions, including trading their Atlanta mansion for a house half its size.[2] Salwen's journey started when his fourteen-year-old daughter saw a homeless man in their upscale neighborhood just a moment before seeing a $100,000 Mercedes pass by. If that person owned a less expensive car, she realized, the homeless man could have a meal. Salwen knew he couldn't redirect someone else's spending and lifestyle choices to remedy this economic disparity. But he could change his own.

The Salwen family generated $800,000 in proceeds from their home-and-possessions sale and donated it to poverty relief work in sub-Saharan Africa. Releasing half their possessions and shifting their focus toward giving infused their family's life with meaning and connection.

I read the Salwens' story around the time I was determined to declutter the kitchen. "Half of this could equal a more meaningful life and a more connected family," I thought. Because I was a stay-at-home mom, the kitchen was like my office. Every dirty dish, every gadget, every crumb-covered counter was like another email in my inbox.

But what if I had less of it to do? What if I had *half* of it to do?

"My goal is no longer to get more done, but to have less to do," writes author Francine Jay in *Miss Minimalist*.[3]

Less to do. Half to do.

Could having half the work make the kitchen table a place of connection again? If I weren't distracted by a looming pile of dishes in the background as I conversed with my husband and kids at dinner, would I be more present? If post-meal cleanup required half the time and energy, would I be freed to journal, read, or take a walk?

I could borrow my kitchen-decluttering strategy from the Salwens' story. I could harness the power of half.

Set Your Intention

A recent poll found that Americans spend an average of sixty-seven minutes per day in their kitchens. That's the equivalent of over four hundred hours (or sixteen days) annually.[4] Of course, this varies based on vocation and life choices. For example, my grandmother (the coffee-shop-phone-call one, not the shopper) spent most of her days in the kitchen while raising nine children.

You likely spend a fair amount of time in your kitchen too, so how do you want it to look and function? What is your intention for this space? Journal it out or jot down a couple of poignant sentences. Ask the Holy Spirit to help you solidify this vision.

Post the paper with your vision of the room's purpose somewhere you'll see it while decluttering (like the microwave).

Pre-Decluttering Work

Before decluttering the kitchen, do these three things:

1. First, toss any trash you find. Focusing on the trash first hones your vision. You're better able to see the

room with new eyes and notice things your brain usually overlooks.

2. Next, remove anything not kitchen-related from the space.

3. Then grab the tools you'll need: several boxes and four baskets (one for water bottles, one for under-the-sink items, one for paper, and one to serve as a clutter catcher).

Declutter Your Kitchen

There are two methods of kitchen decluttering that use the power of half: the quick, ruthless way or the methodical, ruthless way.

You have to be ruthless to make the real change you're being called to. Remember, there is *so much life* on the other side of all your stuff.

QUICK AND RUTHLESS: Grab several boxes and bring them to your kitchen. Place half of the kitchen contents in them. (I like to do this by category: If you have fourteen coffee mugs, narrow it down to seven.) Most of you can do this in an hour. Tell yourself you're simply experimenting with less and not making real decisions yet. This mindset will help you make faster decisions.

Store the boxes away for three months. If you need—truly need—anything from a box during that time, feel free to retrieve it. (Maybe you need more than six forks?) Whatever you didn't need from those boxes during that time, you likely won't ever need. So donate those items.

METHODICAL AND RUTHLESS: Grab a box and dedicate twenty minutes a day to decluttering the following twelve areas, in any order. Again, when the box is full, store it out of sight for three months. Go at it for six days, rest on Sunday, and then continue the next week if needed.

Things You Drink From

Designate a shelf for glasses and a shelf for coffee mugs. Reduce the number to half the original, but also keep only what fits comfortably on the shelf—go past the halfway point if you have to; be daring and dabble with keeping only a third, if needed.

Pile all your water bottles and to-go drink containers in one cleared space. Have each person in the family choose his or her favorite. The rest? Place them in a basket, clear a space in a lower kitchen cabinet, and store them there. It's an experiment, remember. If you need more, bring one back. Storing them in lower cabinets frees your upper cabinets and gives them an uncluttered, unified look upon opening.

Consider swapping your glasses for multifunctional mason jars. These jars can be used as drinking glasses, vases, and food storage containers (think sliced veggies or fruits, soups, etc.). When one item serves multiple purposes, you require fewer possessions.

Utensils, Gadgets, and Silverware

Kitchen gadgets promise to make our lives easier. The spiralizers, graters, shredders, choppers, mixers—each is specific to its own food type. But many of them contribute to clutter. Any pineapple slicing, avocado peeling, or strawberry hulling can easily be done with a knife. An uncluttered kitchen contains tools that serve multiple purposes (like the knife) instead of excess gadgets that serve only one purpose (like the strawberry huller).

For silverware, keep half the number of knives, forks, spoons, and serving spoons. Try it—you can always add some back in.

Plates, Bowls, and Glasses

Wondering how many plates, bowls, and glasses to keep? One to two per person living in your home. If you host regularly and need an extra dish set, store it on the highest shelf, out of everyday use. If too many dishes are in the daily mix, then your kitchen maintenance system (see the "Systems" section on p. 103) won't flow.

Storage Containers

Keep half the number of storage containers (let go of all plastic ones, since some can leach chemicals when heated[5]). Stack the containers inside each other (think Russian-nesting-doll style) to save space. If possible, store the lids in a kitchen drawer for a cleaner look and easy access.

Items for Special Occasions (China, Wineglasses)

China and glasses for special occasions can cross into "sentimental item" territory. (More on this in chapter 12.) Give wine glasses and china each their own high shelf in a kitchen cabinet. Drink tea from the china daily (have tea parties with your children, whatever their age). Sip smoothies and sparkling water from the wine glasses. In the words of writer Ann Wells, "Don't ever save anything for a special occasion. Every day you're alive is a special occasion."[6] If you own it, use it—we're only promised today.

Appliances

The hard-and-fast rule on appliances is to keep the ones you actually use. You can let go of any appliances bought for your aspirational self (the person you once thought you might be but actually aren't). If you're not juicing regularly, jettison the juicer. If the Instant Pot is being used solely as a pantry step stool, find it a new home.

The Front of Your Refrigerator

Remember the UCLA study mentioned in chapter 1 that showed our current society has accumulated the most possessions in the history of time, leaving us stressed? It also found a direct relationship between the amount of stuff covering a refrigerator and the amount of clutter in a home. Researchers, who studied thirty-two Los Angeles homes over a four-year span, found that the average home had fifty-two objects on the fridge's surface. Homes with higher fridge density also had more clutter in the home.[7]

Keep a minimal number of items on the front of your refrigerator, or better yet, clear it entirely. Reducing visual stimuli will make your kitchen feel calmer and may even serve as an impetus for decluttering other areas of your home. Think uncluttered fridge front, uncluttered home, uncluttered soul. It's all related.

Pantry

Pantries become hideouts for expired items. Retrieve them from the recesses of your cabinets, bring them into the light, and toss them. If your kitchen pantry is overstocked, consider donating half its contents to a food bank or shelter.

Try buying just what you need for each week. An emergency kit or backup (stored) pantry can be prudent, especially if you live in an area prone to natural disasters. But stock up from a place of planning and wisdom, not fear.

You don't need to have a perfect pantry, just one that works for you.

Once you have what you want to keep, create a system. Grab baskets or wooden crates and create homes for your items. Sidenote: Home organization is a $12 billion industry. While elevating your home environment and making it beautiful is important, it can cross into unchecked consumerism. For organizational bins, shop your own home first. Can you decorate shoeboxes or unearth a basket from storage? If not, check your local thrift store. You don't have to splurge to have an organized pantry. For an in-depth read on pantry organization, grab Shira Gill's book *Minimalista*.

Junk Drawer

Can you remember what's in this drawer without opening it? If not, then it's likely you don't need most of it. Grab a trash bag and pitch those insignificant contents. Turn your junk drawer into a utility drawer by keeping just what you need. No more searching the house for tape or scissors!

Under the Kitchen Sink

Place a basket under the kitchen sink to hold a bottle of cleaning spray, dish soap, and a dish wand (and bottle brush, depending on the season of life you're in). For an uncluttered look, return these items to the basket after use, and keep only hand soap on the counter.

Counter Spaces

Remember high school physics? Me neither. But I do recall that tightly packed molecules in a high-pressure area rush to spacious, lower pressure areas. Clear countertops are this open, lower pressure, catch-all area; they are a spacious zone liable to attract most anything and everything—keys, purses, papers, random toys, and accessories.

Now that you've removed half of your possessions from the previous categories, hopefully everything fits in the cabinets and your countertops can be clear. In the following Systems section, you'll see how to keep counter spaces clutter free.

Store small appliances (coffeemaker, toaster) out of sight and return each one to its home immediately after using it. The convenience fallacy is the misconception that when we leave items out for later use, our lives become easier. We believe we're simplifying life and saving time—it will be much easier to toast bread if the toaster is already sitting on the counter. The problem is, we only need the toaster for four minutes; the other twenty-three hours and fifty-six minutes of the day, it sits there unused, taking up space and cluttering your countertop. Scan your countertop for appliances that "live" there in hopes of making your life easier, and give them new, hidden homes.

Be sure to have a designated "home" within your home for all bags, jackets, hats, and purses. Return these items to their assigned spot after use (and teach your kids to do the same) or they may gravitate to the kitchen counters.

Systems

No matter how much you own, kitchens, unfortunately, don't have an automatic reset button. The kitchen will stay clutter free only if you implement kitchen-maintenance systems. Thankfully, you need only two: a dishes routine and strategically placed clutter catchers. With less stuff, these systems will finally be manageable.

> **THE DISHES ROUTINE:** At the end of the day, run the dishwasher. Then unload it first thing in the morning. Throughout the day, any dirty dishes go straight into the empty dishwasher (not the sink). If you run out of clean dishes or utensils, grab them from the dishwasher and hand-wash them. After dinner, all dirty dishes are in the dishwasher and the dishwasher is started. Try it. You'll love it!
>
> **CLUTTER CATCHERS:** Place a small basket in your kitchen cabinet (ours is by our plates and bowls). Throughout the day, as random objects appear on the countertops, place them in this basket. Whenever the basket's full, return the "caught" items to their home or place them

in your to-be-donated bag (I call this my "What if we didn't own this?" bag—more on this in chapter 14).

For items that are intentionally placed on the kitchen counter daily, like keys or wallets, ask family members to place them in an aesthetically pleasing, closed container that stays on the counter and hides the clutter. Consider placing the containers where the items are dropped to create a system that simply reshapes an already occurring behavior.

Paper

Paper clutter often infiltrates the heart of the home, piled high on kitchen counters or stuffed away in drawers, even rendering them unopenable. As digital as our world has become, paper is still unavoidable. You likely handle more paper than you think. The average American home still processes a paper stack as high as a two-story house every year.[8]

In her book *The Paper Solution*, Lisa Woodruff recommends the following process to regain control of the paper in your home:

1. **THE BIG PURGE.** Designate a workspace specifically for paper decluttering. Set up five boxes labeled as follows: to sort, to save, to shred, to recycle, and to trash.

   Grab papers from their usual homes (so you see them in a new light) and place them in the "to sort" box. Then handle each piece of paper and ask yourself, "Should I keep this?" If yes, place it in the "to save" box. If no, then place it in the to shred, to recycle, or to trash box. Woodruff proposes that 85 percent of all the paper we have in our lives can be either recycled or shredded.

2. **THE SUNDAY BASKET.** Once you've decluttered your paper, implement the Sunday basket system to keep paper clutter from returning. Take a basket and make that your designated place for any papers around your home that are still active—bills, receipts, letters, notes to yourself, coupons. Any paper that enters your home that isn't immediately recycled is put into this basket. This basket eliminates the piles that form around your house and on your kitchen counters. Plus, you'll always know where to find a paper when needed.

   Find a time on the weekend when you can sit down with the basket and go through the paper items, addressing each item as needed (file, shred, recycle). Try to go through the basket at the same time each week (I choose Saturday afternoon). In Woodruff's experience, this habit takes about six weeks to form. (I keep our basket out of sight in a low kitchen cabinet, but you may choose to keep it on the counter while developing this system.)

3. **MAKE YOUR BINDERS.** Most papers from your "to save" box in Step #1 and papers that are no longer active but still need to be kept and referenced should be put into binders. Woodruff recommends using slash pocket folders to hold your paper within the binders. She doesn't advocate owning a filing cabinet because they allow you to store more paper than you actually need. Woodruff says 90 percent of filing cabinets could be replaced with the following binders: household

reference binder (e.g., warranties, manuals, insurance paperwork), household operations binder (e.g., car, pet, and travel information), financial binder, medical binder, and school memory binder. You can also scan any important documents that you want to save digitally at this point. Once you set up your binder system, some papers will still need to be archived (birth certificates, social security cards, tax returns, passports, etc.). You can use a home safe, a safe deposit box, or an accordion file to archive important papers.

Maintain your systems by going through your Sunday basket weekly and decluttering your binders four times a year, with every season. For more guidance and inspiration on decluttering paper, I highly recommend Woodruff's book *The Paper Solution*.

Finding Peace

Perhaps more than any other room in the house, a cluttered kitchen can be a source of deep restlessness. The antidote to restlessness is peace, and prayer is a tool to promote peace. Peace isn't found in your next purchase or possession but by plugging in to God's presence within you.

Jacques Philippe, in *Searching for and Maintaining Peace*, writes that a heart at peace parallels a calm body of water.[9] For example, when a lake is turbulent, it can't reflect any light. But a calm lake clearly reflects the beauty of the sun's light to everyone who passes. Similarly, a heart at peace allows us to reflect the Son's light to others. Prayer smooths the erratic beats of our heart; it's one way to find that peace.

Jesus often entered prayer by retreating to the mountains, the wilderness, or other solitary places. Entering a quiet place to pray wasn't a one-time thing—it was a top priority for Jesus, the defining rhythm of his life.

"When we pray, genuinely pray, the real condition of our heart is revealed," writes Richard Foster in his book *Prayer: Finding the Heart's True Home.* "This is as it should be. This is when God truly begins to work with us. The adventure is just beginning."[10]

The same is true for us. Without prayer, we can't truly know God or make space for him to work in our hearts. Without prayer, we are left unfulfilled, with a restless inner itch for more.

In my journey toward minimalism, I found inner calm in prayer. The feeling was novel and fleeting at first, but after I sensed it, I wanted more. The mornings when I entered into God's presence at my kitchen table led to mornings laced with more peace and, eventually, to moments throughout the day when I would realize he was there with me.

My physical space was part of this spiritual journey. The kitchen's outer calm supported an inner calm and a newfound space for solitude and space for Jesus, who alone is Peace.

---

10 Items to Declutter from Your Kitchen

When decluttering the kitchen categories mentioned in this chapter, be sure to remove the following items:

1. Extra coffee mugs
2. Spatulas (Do you really need five of them? Try living with only one for a month and see.)

3. Food storage containers with missing or broken lids
4. Old medicines or vitamins
5. Plastic shopping bags (get reusable ones)
6. Expired food or freezer-burned food
7. Stale pantry items
8. Expired spices
9. Cookbooks you never use (bookmark online recipes instead)
10. Takeout menus (you can find them online)

Inner Decluttering Tool: Create Your Quiet Place

Our hearts are designed to rest in God. Here's how to create a quiet place to meet with him:

- Designate an area of your home to be your "meeting place" with Jesus. Maybe it's your kitchen table, a chair in your bedroom, or even your closet floor.
- Commit to meeting Jesus there in silence at the same time each day. (Consider starting a prayer journal and recording the inspirations he gives you during this quiet time.)

Prayer opens the door to our inner home, opening our heart to his presence. Show up for this meeting daily.

Outer Decluttering Tool: Declutter the Front of the Fridge

As mentioned, the amount of stuff you place on your fridge likely reflects the amount of clutter in your home. If you want to take immediate action and make your kitchen feel lighter in minutes, declutter the front of your fridge.

- Remove magnets.
- File papers.
- Rehome written reminders.
- Relocate photos (or just display your favorite).

Now, whenever you see the clear fridge, let the drastic change remind you that the rest of your home is about to undergo a similar transformation. You are creating a clutter-free life.

CHAPTER

9

DECLUTTERING YOUR WARDROBE AND LETTING GO OF COMPARISON

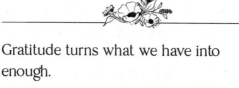

Gratitude turns what we have into enough.

—ANONYMOUS

The seeds of my wardrobe preoccupation were sown in early childhood while perusing sale racks with Grandma, observing her overflowing closets, and, ultimately, concluding that the newest trends and styles were a measuring stick for self-worth.

Around the time I entered high school, I realized that the opportunities for wardrobe-based social comparison were ubiquitous. Seeing someone dressed in a trendy, popular outfit would trigger an impetuous examination of my outfit of choice and, indirectly, my self-worth. Was my outfit trendier than theirs or did it tout more brand names? If so, then I felt good, accepted. If not, I immediately felt bad. And unless the color just wasn't me (think pale yellow), I instantly wanted what they had.

Even in high school, I knew what Jesus would have to say about this. In fact, if we had met up at the corner coffee shop where I used to "borrow" friends' calculus assignments, this likely would have been his greeting: "Why do you worry about clothes?" (Matthew 6:28).

But the Dr. Martens boots? I needed them. And the silver hoop earrings and the bling Gadzooks belt? Life wasn't complete—and I wasn't content—until I wore them. I even began documenting my wardrobe combinations to ensure I wouldn't repeat the same ensemble twice in one month. Soon I could recite outfit combinations—my own and those of others—more fluently than any anatomy lesson or bit of assigned Shakespeare.

While wardrobes can be a form of self-expression, this outfit preoccupation went beyond simply conveying an outward sign of "me." This was social comparison at its finest. My preoccupation trailed close behind as I entered college and the work world, leaving in its wake a closet overflowing with outfits purchased in an attempt to bolster my self-worth.

With the rise of advertising and social media, more people struggle with comparison today than ever. But comparison evaporates joy. God hasn't called humans to have hearts of comparison, but rather to "test their own actions . . . without comparing themselves to someone else" (Galatians 6:4).

Comparison delivers the feeling that, to use the words of French poet Arthur Rimbaud, "the real life is elsewhere."[1] If your life constantly fails to "measure up," then you focus on the negatives of your situation and the things you lack. This begets discouragement, envy, and the perpetual itch to buy more. In looking at the lives of others, in believing the real life is elsewhere, you often forget to live.

Your wardrobe is an opportunity to either reflect your true self to the world or constantly compare yourself to it and then strive to conform. Decluttering it is one important part of finding inner contentment.

Minimizing your wardrobe, shedding social comparison, and fighting the urge to refill empty hangers with sale items allows you to focus on the unchanging and unseen. It provides space for God to affirm your authentic self—the person he created a certain way, for a specific reason.

An Obsession with the Visible

Curating an authentic wardrobe, free from outside influence, means accepting Gabrielle Bossis's challenge to her readers: "May the invisible be more present to you than the visible."[2]

Yet today's fashion industry capitalizes on our obsession with the visible. In 1930 the average woman had 36 items in her closet—today it's 120.[3] Most fashion trends today last around two to four months, placing consumers in a constant purchasing spiral as they attempt to keep up.[4] Our planet, pocketbooks, and stress levels are bearing the costs of fast fashion and elusive trends.

Consider the following ecological statistics from Shannon Lohr, who trains entrepreneurs to build sustainable fashion businesses through her online program Factory45:[5]

- The amount of water used in apparel production each year is enough to fill thirty-two million Olympic-sized swimming pools. (Meanwhile, 2.2 billion people lack access to safe drinking water.)[6]
- By extending the life of their clothing an additional nine months, the average consumer could reduce their carbon, waste, and water footprints by 20 to 30 percent each.
- Clothing made from conventional polyester can take two hundred years to decompose in a landfill.
- Making a pair of jeans uses the same amount of water as flushing your toilet for three years.

The average American household spends $160 on clothing each month (nearly $2,000 a year),[7] but studies show we wear only 20 percent of our clothing.[8] And yet 61 percent of Americans regularly stand before their full closets and claim they have "nothing to wear."[9]

What's the remedy to our textile overconsumption and discontent?

The Capsule Wardrobe

The solution to fast fashion–filled closets is simply less. Less purchasing on impulse, less accumulating from envy, less believing every tantalizing good deal is a "need," and less consumption of cheaply made clothing.

Enter the capsule wardrobe. Sound familiar? I'd consider it a buzzword in the minimalism world, made even more popular by Courtney Carver's book *Project 333: The Minimalist Fashion Challenge That Proves Less Really Is So Much More.*

A capsule wardrobe is a wardrobe composed of inter-changeable pieces that greatly simplify the decision of what to wear. In short, most everything "goes" together—the minimal but matching clothing items yield many outfit combos.

The premise of Carver's *Project 333* is simply this: Wear just 33 items for 3 months. All clothing, accessories, jewelry, outerwear, and shoes count toward your number. Exceptions include wedding rings, underwear, sleepwear, in-home lounge-wear, and workout clothing.

By simplifying your wardrobe, Carver says, you will "get back all the joy you were missing while you were worrying about what to wear."[10]

Her advice was the start of my journey away from outfit preoccupation and toward authenticity. I realized that a cap-sule wardrobe could mean freedom from comparison. It could allow me to reclaim joy in the way I expressed myself to the world.

It can do the same for you too.

How to Create a Capsule Wardrobe You Love

1. DISCERN YOUR STYLE

The first step to creating a capsule wardrobe you love is know-ing what you love to wear. Not what you think you "should" wear, but what outfits, when worn, carry zero feelings of unease because they make you feel like you. What is your favorite outfit and why? What outfits are most flattering on you? What outfits and colors do you feel your best in?

Hang up one of your favorite outfits so it's visible while you declutter. This is your gold standard—run every outfit by this beloved one. Aim to keep only the outfits that you love as much as this one. You want every single outfit in your closet to be a favorite that fits your current lifestyle.

Discerning a style that you love can also involve deepening your self-love. To quote Carver, "You'll never find something to wear that makes you feel beautiful, smart, and loved if you don't believe you already are."[11]

2. DECLUTTER FOR WHO YOU ARE TODAY

Once you've determined your favorite style, it's time to declutter your wardrobe. Take every piece of clothing out of your closet, drawers, and storage and pile it all onto your bed. (If you are short on time or expect interruptions, then declutter by clothing category—shorts one day, T-shirts the next, etc. This way if you need to stop midproject, you won't be dressing from piles of clothes on your floor all week.)

Brace yourself—the clothing pile might be massive. Mine was. When I saw my pile, the anonymous quote "All that clutter used to be money" came to mind. *All that clothing used to be money.* I decided instead to focus on the words of Cassandra Aarssen, author of *Real Life Organizing*: "Remember that the money you spent on that item is gone. You're not any richer if you store this item in your home, and you won't be any poorer if you let it go."[12]

Take a couple of deep breaths if you need to, pump some upbeat music, and place a "comfort item" nearby (like a favorite tea or sparkling water). Now dive in. Hold every clothing item, inspect it, and decide if it is worthy of your new capsule wardrobe. If yes, hang it back up. If no, throw it on the floor. You may want to create a third pile for favorite items that are out of season. You can hang your off-season items in your closet if you'd like access to them year-round (cozy sweaters can be useful in an overly air-conditioned office) or store them separately (as seen in step #3).

Only keep wardrobe items that support who you are today. Keep some maternity clothes if you plan to have more kids, but let go of the jeans you're hoping to fit into someday. They can make you feel like you're not enough today. Dressing for someone you used to be or for a future "aspirational self" will distract you from your life, cement you in I'll-be-happier-when thought patterns, and cause you to miss out on who you are today. In the words of John Mark Comer, "The [present] moment is where you find God, find your soul, find your life."[13]

If you're battling the urge to keep wardrobe items "just in case," then review the tools in chapter 6 to help shift your mindset. Also, if you need more than intuition to declutter your wardrobe, try The Minimalists' 90/90 rule.[14] Hold an item and ask, "Have I used this in the last 90 days? Will I use it in the next 90 days?" If you answered no to both questions, give yourself permission to let it go and bless someone else who needs it.

Pay attention to each article of clothing you choose to declutter. Why are you letting it go (was it the fit, the colors, etc.)? Use this information to make better clothing purchases in the future.

---

3. DONATE OR BOX UP EXTRA CLOTHES

After hanging up items you're keeping, address the piles of clothing lining the floor of your bedroom. Separate them into two piles: save and donate. You may choose to save several off-season items, a couple of maternity outfits, and pieces that you're not yet prepared to part with but know you may part with later. Transfer the save pile to a storage bin. Set a reminder on your phone to revisit the bin in three months. By that time, any on-the-fence items that you haven't needed you can confidently let go.

Next, address the donate pile. Fill multiple boxes with the items that no longer fit your lifestyle. Be prepared for intense feelings that may arise during this step. Never-worn items still bearing price tags may trigger guilt or shame. An inner voice prompting, "But what if I need that someday?" may trigger fear. Handling the black dress you wore to your grandma's funeral will likely trigger sadness.

Acknowledge every feeling, feel every feeling, thank every feeling for showing up, and then tell it you no longer have need of it or its associated textile trigger. Now donate the boxes and release the weight of negative feelings that have been packed away in your closet. By choosing to own only the items you love, you're inviting positivity into your life each time you open your closet.

4. Create the Capsule

Assess the items that made the initial cut and are now hanging in your closet. You can assign a set number of clothing items to retain, or you can go with your intuition. Our lives aren't the same, so no arbitrary "right amount" of clothing exists. If you want more structure, count out thirty-three items and join Carver's minimalist challenge. She recommends decluttering your wardrobe four times a year, as the seasons change. Setting up a thirty-three-piece capsule wardrobe for each season doesn't mean keeping 132 items (4 x 33), 99 of which stay in storage. When you're creating a new capsule, assess the items from the previous season and find crossover pieces.[15] One pair of jeans can be worn in winter, spring, and fall. The same black T-shirt dress can be worn year-round, just add leggings and a cardigan for fall and winter. A basic white V-neck tee can be worn in every season. Focusing on crossover pieces will help reduce the size of your overall wardrobe.

To curate a capsule wardrobe, keep clothing items that are in line with your lifestyle and your clothing style. The key is to mix and match flattering staples to create a simple, versatile, sustainable wardrobe you love. It may help to choose primarily neutral colors, plus one or two colors you love to wear. Then add more variety and color with a few key accessories.

If you can't decide what items to pick, start with this formula and modify as you go:[16]

4 pairs of shoes
2 bags (purse, tote, etc.)
1 pair of sunglasses
1 scarf
3 pieces of jewelry
2 coats/jackets
2 dresses or skirts (if you wear dresses or skirts)
3 pairs of pants (if you wear pants)
10 tops (shirts/sweaters)

5. Skip Unnecessary Shopping

Creating a capsule wardrobe is not an excuse to go shopping. Use what you have, or if needed, add only a couple of items.

Be mindful of the Diderot effect as you declutter

accessories and shoes. The Diderot effect occurs when purchasing one item creates a "need" to purchase more items.[17]
For example, you buy a new shirt, so suddenly you need new
shoes, a new necklace, and a new purse to match. Normally
you wouldn't have purchased those accessories, but since you
bought the shirt, one purchase led to another. If you decide
to declutter the shirt that started the purchasing spiral, then
you can let go of the matching shoes, necklace, and purse too.

6. ROCK YOUR WARDROBE AND OBSERVE

The lightness you will feel when scanning your newly decluttered closet will be immediate. I began mixing and matching
outfits each morning and soon found I loved the simplicity and
also the creativity involved. The wardrobe I had compiled was
working for me.

Carver recommends sticking with your set wardrobe for
three months to truly test whether a capsule wardrobe is for
you. During this time, observe what it's like to have a simplified
wardrobe full of only flattering pieces you love. Is your stress
level lower in the morning when deciding what to wear? Do you
save time getting dressed in the morning? Is your self-talk more
positive because you consistently like how you look? Are you
less inclined to shop since you love what you already own?

Be prepared to repeat outfits. No one cares if you wear
the same thing twice in a week, or even on consecutive
days. Research shows that, after each interaction,
people spend only about ten seconds thinking about
you; they're usually thinking about themselves.[18]

Less Decision Fatigue

When deciding what to wear involves sorting through crammed closets and umpteen wardrobe options, our brains can become fatigued before the day even begins. *Decision fatigue*, a term first coined by social psychologist Dr. Roy Baumeister in his research at Florida State University, simply means the more decisions we make, the more difficult making our next decision becomes.[19] Baumeister discovered that humans have a finite amount of daily willpower that wears away as we make decisions.

Think of it this way. Our decision-making power source is like our phone battery. We start out the day at 100%, but as the day goes on and we make decisions, our mental charge depletes.

Do I hit snooze or get up with my alarm? Down to 99%.

Do I make the bed? 98%

Do I check my phone or do quiet time first? 97%

Do I wear this, or this, or this, or this? 93%

And so the decision-making continues into our day.

Some are easy: "Mom, can I jump off the kitchen table and show how I fly?" ("Um, absolutely not—get down now!") Down to 65%.

Or more weighted: Do we send our first grader to school this year or homeschool? Down to 40%.

With every decision made, our decision-making reserve decreases. When our battery gets low (could be by noon, depending on the day), so does our willpower and ability to make good decisions.

Minimizing your wardrobe reduces the number of outfit

options you must consider. While you don't have to take it as far as Mark Zuckerberg, who basically owns duplicates of one outfit, great minds like his are onto something. By minimizing your wardrobe, you also minimize the number of morning decisions you have to make, saving your decision-making power for more important choices later in the day.

Overcoming Social Comparison

As I became more confident in my personal style, I began observing, and liking, what others wore without coveting their wardrobe items. I noticed that the nagging inner voice—the one telling me I should wear what others were wearing—was growing quieter. But it took more than just a decluttered wardrobe to render it silent.

I needed the deeper antidote to social comparison: gratitude.

Thankfulness is essential to your inner decluttering journey too. Just as your outer world is simplified by a curated capsule wardrobe, your inner world is simplified by replacing your comparing heart with a grateful one that's thankful for not only what you own but also who you are.

The theme of thanksgiving is plastered all over the New Testament. Paul's prolific writings focus not on accumulating more but on being thankful for the gifts you already have. Consider his letter to the Colossians:

> So then, just as you received Christ Jesus as Lord, continue to live your lives in him, rooted and built up in him, strengthened in the faith as you were taught, and overflowing with thankfulness. (Colossians 2:6–7)

Let the peace of Christ rule in your hearts, since as members of one body you were called to peace. And be thankful. (Colossians 3:15)

Whatever you do, whether in word or deed, do it all in the name of the Lord Jesus, giving thanks to God the Father through him. (Colossians 3:17)

It's through gratitude—and only gratitude—that we realize life is a gift. It is *the practice* of thankfulness that allows you to stop looking outside yourself for contentment. When you're aware that your source of joy resides within you, your heart can develop a Psalm 23 posture: "There is nothing I lack" (v. 1 NABRE).

God is the giver of all things good in our lives. When the gifts eclipse the Giver, when we focus on stuff instead of its source, comparison sets in. To quote Paul again, "What do you have that you did not receive?" (1 Corinthians 4:7). Read that again. An unseen force is at work in your life, sustaining your every breath, providing for your every need.

God's goodness and presence are within you, around you, covering your life—the life you have, not the life you wish you had, expected to have, or feel you deserve to have. Can you see that? Is your heart in tune with his gifts?

It's taken years for my eyes to see his gifts daily and for my heart to shift toward gratitude. I started documenting moments I'm grateful for in 2015, after reading Ann Voskamp's book *One Thousand Gifts*. Her book is where I learned that gratitude is simply a matter of focus.

My gratitude journal now has thousands of entries—moments

that continue to fill me with joy that I otherwise would have overlooked or forgotten: A beautiful sunset. Big brown toddler eyes looking over a strawberry ice cream bar. My husband's jokes. Being told, "Mama, thank you for taking good care of me," at 3:00 a.m. My favorite NEEDTOBREATHE song on the radio. A quality phone conversation with my mom during nap time. Family strolls on stunning fall Sundays.

These recordings have shown me that the things I'm most thankful for aren't tangible things at all.

An intentional shift toward gratitude has changed how I see the world. It can do the same for you. Gratitude won't make you always happy—that's not real life. It will, however, make your life simpler and more joy-filled as you carve out more space for contentment with who you are and what you have.

---

10 Things to Declutter from Your Wardrobe

1. Shoes you don't like or that hurt your feet
2. Clothing you don't think you will wear again

Change the direction of your hanger once you wear a piece of clothing and hang it back up. By the end of the month, see what hangers haven't flipped the opposite direction. If you haven't worn these items in a month, do you still need them?

---

3. Purses you don't use
4. Clothes with the tags still attached
5. Clothes that don't fit who you are today
6. Clothes unable to be repaired
7. Any items that make you sad or guilty

8. Clothes other people gifted you that you don't love
9. That one-time-wear formal outfit
10. Underwear and socks with holes

Inner Decluttering Tool: Adopt a Gratitude Practice

Where is the goodness of God in your life today? Even during inevitable seasons of lament, God's hand is at work. He will accompany you through them. There is always something to be thankful for—every breath is a gift.

Choose one of the following gratitude practices and start it today. (As you begin, consider placing a visual cue like a notecard that reads "Give Thanks" somewhere you will see it often.) Once you have one of these "mastered," add another one.

- Record three things you're thankful for each night in a gratitude journal (a study out of the University to San Diego found that eight weeks of gratitude journaling can literally improve cardiac function).[20]
- Anytime you catch your heart moving toward comparison, counter that by immediately thinking of three things you're grateful for.
- At family dinner, go around the table and have each family member say one thing they are thankful for.

- When you're stopped at a red light, pause and thank God for one thing.
- On Sunday evening after dinner, have each family member reflect on one thing they are grateful for from the past week.
- Express gratitude to God daily for how he created you. He's made you a specific way to help you fulfill your God-given mission during your brief time on earth. Reflect on what you love about yourself and tell him thanks.

Outer Decluttering Tool: Find Your Personal Style

Again, the first step to creating a capsule wardrobe is developing your personal style. Here's the nitty-gritty on how to navigate that first step:

11. Create a T-chart with the word *Love* on the right and *Don't love* on the left.
12. Now look through recent photos of yourself and record each outfit in one of the categories. Tap into your Inner Guide; how does each outfit make you feel? What type of self-talk arises? (For example, if a photo of yourself in a blue A-line dress conveys an expansive, light feeling or inner dialogue like, "I really love that dress," then write "blue A-line dress" in the "Love" category).

13. Look for trends in the "Love" category. Do blue items keep showing up? Are graphic tees your thing?
14. Below the T-chart write a line or two summing up your personal clothing style. (For example, "The clothing I love and feel my best in has either a unique, artsy quality to it or a graphic that articulates a meaningful message. All pieces must be amazingly comfortable.")
15. Tape your chart to your bathroom mirror and memorize it before decluttering your closet. When you know your personal style, letting go becomes much easier.

If you didn't record enough items in the "Love" category to observe trends or if you want a more objective resource, then google "Stitch Fix Body Calculator." With a few measurements, you can determine your body type and the styles that best suit you.

For an in-depth dive into wardrobe decluttering, I highly recommend Carver's book *Project 333*.

10

DECLUTTERING THE LIVING ROOM / BEDROOM AND LETTING GO OF HURRY

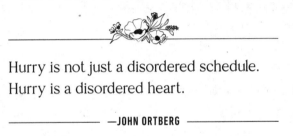

Hurry is not just a disordered schedule.
Hurry is a disordered heart.

—JOHN ORTBERG

Around the time I turned my decluttering efforts to the living room and bedroom, a particular phrase kept popping up: "Jesus pace." A repeat thought is often a sign that the Holy Spirit is trying to tell me something. And by the fourth or fifth time, he's usually grabbed my attention.

A Jesus pace. Wasn't it his mission and love that mattered? Why the sudden prompting to ponder the speed at which he moved throughout his earthly ministry?

The answer hit me like a freight train on a chaotic morning while I was trying to get kids to preschool on time. The clock was ticking, my self-perceived pressure was growing, and soon

I was barking orders and ricocheting around the home in a this-is-not-at-all-how-I-want-to-parent fashion.

A Jesus pace. In my soul, I heard the inner prompting. And I finally understood: Jesus was *never* in a hurry.

Yet hurry was my baseline—one that made my life a blur of constant movement, unholy rushing, and contrived urgency. I often found myself holding my breath—cutting off my very life source—in fear of what might happen if I stopped, arrived late, or didn't get enough done. I was hyperliving, yes. But rushing wasn't truly living. At my frenetic pace I was, at best, skimming the surface of my one life.

Psalm 39:6 (NLT) says, "We are merely moving shadows, and all our busy rushing ends in nothing." A life full of movement, yet vapid, void.

In *The Rest of God*, Mark Buchanan writes, "I cannot think of a single advantage I've ever gained from being in a hurry. But a thousand broken and missed things, tens of thousands, lie in the wake of the rushing. . . . Through all that haste I thought I was *making up time*. It turns out I was *throwing it away*."[1]

Jesus never worried about time. Maybe because his perception of time involved eternity—time without end. And he extends that promise to those who are his. I was promised eternity, but I still felt like I never had enough time.

I was starting to see the problem more clearly. Hurry closed the door of the soul, cut off the connection with the Father, and numbed the movements of the Spirit. In the words of Ann Voskamp, "The hurry makes us hurt."[2]

Thomas Merton agreed by calling "the rush and pressure of modern life" a "pervasive form of contemporary violence."[3]

Hurt. Violence. No wonder medical professionals have now coined the term "hurry sickness" as a treatable condition in our culture. Meyer Friedman, a cardiologist, first documented the phrase after noticing that the majority of his at-risk cardiovascular patients presented with an increased "sense of time urgency."[4]

Hurry is a condition of the heart.

My need to slow down was palpable. Not only because I wanted to emulate Jesus but also because God had commanded his people to remember the Sabbath day.

Writer Corrie ten Boom said that if the devil can't make you sin, he'll make you busy. Read that again. BUSY might as well stand for "being under Satan's yoke." Slowing down is a full-handed slap in the face to the Enemy. Both sin and busyness isolate us from God. They sever the transformative union between us and our Beloved.

I could feel that separation in my own life.

The places of rest within my home beckoned. The gray chaise sofa, the worn recliner, our cozy queen bed—these corners of our home invited me to pause, put up my feet, and dive deeper into the sacred moments of this life. But they were consistently covered in clutter. How could I permit myself to rest if all I saw was more to be done? And how could I, practically speaking, put up my feet if the sofa was crammed with random stuff?

The clutter in these areas was a barrier to accepting the rest they were designed to give. A blanket of extraneous possessions robbed the rooms of any sentiments of rest—again, my inner state on display.

I needed to face my inclination to move through life at an

accelerated pace. But I also needed to clear out the spaces of rest in my home: the living room and bedroom.

Decluttering Spaces of Rest

The living room and bedroom are designed to be spaces for rest and connection. Restoring these spaces to their original purpose allows us to slow down our lives and live more deeply connected to God.

Is God calling you toward a slower, more connected life? If anything you've read so far in this chapter resonates—if simply *imagining* slowing down feels like a deep breath, a lifted weight—then it's likely so. Your environment can set the tone for this pace-based pivot. Here's how.

1. **WHAT IS YOUR VISION?** Before decluttering your living room and bedroom, develop your vision for these rooms. Be specific—we're talking laser-like precision. Let the purpose of these two rooms become so clear that you could outline it in your sleep. Write down a phrase or several words that define your rooms' purpose. I chose *connection* and *rest*. These words were the standard by which every item in the room was measured. If something didn't pass the connection-and-rest test, it didn't stay. Maybe your word is *leisure* or *a space for hobbies* (both forms of rest).

2. **GET THE TRASH OUT FIRST.** Begin decluttering these spaces by culling the trash first. Long-abandoned fruit snack wrappers, unneeded Amazon boxes, forgotten receipts—toss it all. As mentioned before, focusing

on trash first is like a decluttering warm-up: you're making decisions, removing clutter, and beginning to look at the room in a different way. Your momentum is flowing.

3. **RETURN ITEMS TO THEIR PROPER HOMES.** Return any items that don't belong in your living room or bedroom to their proper homes. Disheveled clothes go to the laundry room, the half-eaten bowl of cereal goes to the sink, the little Monopoly dog goes back to the box . . . you get the picture. You want to channel your decluttering efforts to living room and bedroom items only.

4. **BEGIN DECLUTTERING THE REMAINING ITEMS.** Hold each item and ask, "Does this item fit my vision for this space?" Grab a box or trash bag—consider using a black one so what you donate remains out of sight—and ruthlessly pile in whatever doesn't fulfill the room's purpose.

   Call upon your Inner Guide again. You'll know when an item is a 100 percent match with your vision for the room. And you'll know if something is genuinely important to you or not. CDs buried at the bottom of a basket clearly were not that important before you unearthed them, and seeing them again does not redeem their value.

   Maybe you need less furniture, fewer (or no) TVs, fewer knickknack-adorned shelves, or fewer book stacks to better focus on the people in front of you. Remember that most of us use only 20 percent of our stuff. Don't let your mental, spiritual, and physical space be weighed down by the trivial.

5. **DECIDE WHAT TO DO WITH THE BOXED-UP ITEMS.** If you're not

donating items right away, then store your boxes, but for no longer than two to three months. Schedule an "appointment" with yourself for when you'll go through the boxes. Write it on your calendar and set a reminder on your phone.

If you are donating items right away, decide on a charity and pass your old things on to bless someone else. Facebook Buy Nothing groups are another great option for letting go of items. You post a photo of the item, people who need the item comment, and you choose the recipient. This service gives a personal touch to the rehoming of your items.

If you're letting go of large possessions (think furniture) or high-end items, consider selling them. Facebook Marketplace is a popular selling platform.

Use Technology as a Tool

Consider how technology can assist your decluttering. If you can't part with those CDs, could you download them onto your computer or upload them to your phone and still enjoy them? Could you take photos of living room items you want to remember, create a "living room photo album" on your phone, and scroll through them whenever you feel called? Technology can allow us to still enjoy the memory or feeling attached to an item without actually owning it.

Consider Wall Decor

Wall decor in the living room and bedroom is an extension of each room's purpose. When deciding what to keep on your walls, be intentional and don't overdo it. Wall decor creates visual noise. And according to author Josef Pieper, visual noise dampens the soul's ability to perceive spiritual realities.[5]

Just as too many possessions can be distracting, so can too much wall decor. Simply put, "wall clutter" can be stress-inducing and soul-stifling.

William Morris said, "Have nothing in your house that you do not know to be useful or believe to be beautiful."[6] Reflect on what you truly consider beautiful and ask yourself how you feel when you encounter a piece of wall decor. Remove any wall art that you bought just because it was a "good deal" or hung simply to fill white space. (Don't be afraid of white space—studies show it can increase serotonin levels and reduce blood pressure for a calming effect.[7]) The best wall decor is a reflection of you, your family, and your values; it's not a random collection of the best deals you found at Target and T.J.Maxx.

A Note about Books

Books often live in places of rest. It makes sense—books facilitate rest. A 2009 study by the University of Sussex revealed that a mere six minutes of reading can reduce a person's stress level by 68 percent.[8] Been reading this chapter for at least six minutes? Your stress levels may be lower for it.

But holding on to books we don't love, books we've neglected to read, or books we bought for our "aspirational self" can also invoke stress and trigger feelings of guilt. Scan your books for those that bring up a negative feeling and let them go immediately.

Define the physical boundaries where your books will live, and then keep only what fits within these boundaries. This could be one bookcase or one shelf. You can keep as many books as you like, but they can't surpass this designated space. When you get a new book, an old one will have to go (think "one in, one out") to honor the boundary and keep your space clutter free.

Unless you plan to reread a book or reference it often, consider giving it to a friend who might enjoy it. For books you're less attached to, think about donating your copy and checking another one out from the library as needed. (If you regret letting a book go, you can purchase it again for a few dollars at a used bookstore.) For more tips on decluttering books, go to www.richinwhatmatters.com and search "books."

"Remember: you are not what you own," says author Francine Jay. "Storing all those books doesn't make you any smarter; it just makes your life more cluttered."[9]

Closets

Most areas of rest have a closet close by—whether it's a linen closet, bedroom closet, or hall closet. You can use the five-step decluttering tool mentioned previously to realign this space with your original vision for it.

You can also use this five-step tool for decluttering your bathrooms. For an in-depth look at decluttering bathrooms, visit www.richinwhatmatters.com and search "bathroom."

Decide your purpose and vision for the space. Closets aren't designed to be catchalls. How do you want the area to look and function? Write it out so your intention for the space is clear, and come back to it for clarity as needed.

To reset a closet, I like to remove everything from the

closet, wipe it down, and refill it with only essentials. A complete closet clear-out may be more of a project than you have time to conquer in one sitting. You may opt to declutter shelf by shelf or by zones.

There's no wrong method; just choose one and dive in. Remember, this is important work. In the words of author Cheryl Richardson, "If you want to improve your life immediately, clean out a closet. Often it's what we hold onto that holds us back."[10]

Grab your trash bag and remove all trash first. Next, return misplaced items to their proper homes. Now, with your vision firmly in mind, put items back in the closet only if they align with your goal for the closet. Box up the remaining items and work through them either now or in two to three months. If items are sentimental in nature, see chapter 12 for how to declutter these items.

Calendar Clutter

Even if the main living areas of the home are clutter free, if your calendar is still packed, you won't be putting your feet up as planned. So ask yourself, "Is there any calendar clutter I need to remove to make space in my schedule to use this room the way I envisioned?" A shorter version of this question may be, "What do I need to say no to?"

Lysa TerKeurst says, "Whenever you say yes to something, there is less of you for something else. Make sure your yes is worth the less."[11]

Read that again. Saying *yes* to heading the trivia night fundraiser at your kid's school might mean *less* time at home with them. Saying *yes* to an extra project at work might mean *less* energy for your daily duties. So ask yourself, "Is the *yes* worth the *less?*" Remember that when we say no, we give others the opportunity to step up and say yes.

In *Essentialism*, Greg McKeown makes a similar point. He recommends saying yes only if the commitment is something you feel 100 percent called to. He says, "If it isn't a clear yes, then it's a clear no."[12] Note that a *clear* yes doesn't always mean a *comfortable* yes. Could God call us to vacate our comfort zone at times and answer a call that requires full reliance on him? Absolutely.

My favorite tool for deciphering a clear yes is uttering this simple prayer three times: "Come Holy Spirit, come." And then listening to my Inner Guide the best I can. I may not "get it right" every time, but if a decision is rooted in prayer, I trust he will bring something good out of it.

A Slower Pace

Enjoying these newly decluttered spaces of rest requires uprooting hurry from your inner home. It requires a slower pace—a Jesus pace. Start by taking daily mini sabbaths where you devote midday moments to stopping, sitting, and just being with God.

At first you might not know what to do when you aren't, well, *doing*. Slowness, stillness, the antithesis of rushing, can feel awkward and uncomfortable. During these intentional pauses, center yourself through mindfulness activities, like mentally describing your surroundings (include sights, sounds, smells, tastes, and sensations). Then focus on connecting with God.

You can also use grounding techniques to slow down, like

wrapping your hands around a mug of hot tea, taking deep breaths, and inhaling the aroma. Intentional pauses will form a rhythm in your day defined by connection, not rushing.

Watch for your "rushing patterns," and identify the times you feel inclined to rush. Mine often happened when I was about to leave the house, especially if I was running late. Use mantras like "Relationships first" or "The hurry only hurts" as a cue to slow yourself down during triggered times.

For example, I resolved that staying calm in front of our kids (who were immediately triggered if I was) mattered more to me than getting somewhere on time or completing a task quickly. While I couldn't completely eschew punctuality or efficiency, I could move at a pace that supported me, my God-given dignity, and my nervous system.

Begin taking the Sabbath seriously. Don't view it as a catch-up-on-everything day. (Thanks to your decluttering efforts, you're likely beginning to have less to do and more time to enjoy.) Run your Sabbath activities through the rest-or-worship test. Is the activity rest or worship? If the answer is no, then it isn't fit for the Sabbath.

Your new pace, supported by uncluttered spaces of rest, will likely feel right. But any moment holds the power to throw you back into "doing mode"—a child proudly strewing Cheerios across the clutter-free couch, another child getting into the makeup and adorning her arms with eyeliner-based dalmatian spots. But when you practice slow living, you notice the forward shift toward hurry and can remind yourself to lean back into "being mode" instead of automatically jumping from one task to the next. And when you're on top of your game, you can start doing these tasks for God.

For me, slower living felt like deeper living. It was a pace that allowed me to notice life and the Giver of it. A pace that if Jesus came over (and effortlessly grabbed a clear seat) would allow me to sit comfortably at his feet.

---

10 Things to Declutter from Your Living Room

1. Excess bowls/containers/baskets
2. Objects missing parts (like the digital photo frame from ten years ago that you still can't find the cord to)
3. Books you didn't enjoy or never finished reading
4. Broken tools
5. Knickknacks
6. Hobby items you don't use
7. Unused remotes
8. Unused media (DVDs, CDs, video games)
9. Excess furniture
10. Excess decorative pillows

---

10 Things to Declutter from Your Bedroom

1. Unused exercise equipment
2. Burnt-out candles
3. Too many extra linens
4. Piles of paper clutter
5. Old magazines
6. Excess flashlights
7. Anything that doesn't belong (bowls, mugs, markers)

8. Dead plants
9. Random unused cords
10. Old planners or journals

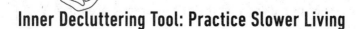

Inner Decluttering Tool: Practice Slower Living

Make your own list of practical ways you can slow down today. We are embodied people, so slowing our actions can also slow our physical heart, which leads to slowing the pace of our inner world. Here are some ideas:

- Walk slowly.
- Sit next to a child for ten minutes and watch them play.
- Practice deep, diaphragmatic breathing (inhale through nose for four seconds, pause briefly, exhale through mouth for six seconds).[13]
- Pencil two to three mini sabbaths into your daily schedule. Make these five- to ten-minute pauses devoted to stopping, sitting, and just being with God.
- Stop fully at a stop sign and drive the speed limit.
- Complete one task at a time instead of multitasking.
- Spend time in nature, simply observing.

Practice two to three of these daily and watch the pace of your life decelerate. Life is all around us, waiting to be lived and enjoyed more deeply.

Outer Decluttering Tool:
Declutter a Space of Rest

Author Brené Brown said, "It takes courage to say yes to rest . . . in a culture where exhaustion is seen as a status symbol."[14] Take a step in a countercultural, life-giving direction by making your main living areas places of rest. Here's how:

- Ask yourself, "Which main living space in my home is causing me the most stress?" Is it the living room, bedroom, or an associated area like the bathroom or your book nook?
- Now use the steps in this chapter to declutter that space and transform it into a true area of rest.

Clear the clutter and watch your heart and life become grounded in rest and calm.

PART 3

Decluttering the Upstairs / Mind

The mind will always take on an order conforming to that upon which it concentrates.

—RICHARD FOSTER

11

DECLUTTERING KIDS' STUFF AND LETTING GO OF REACTIVITY

If you want your children to turn out well,
spend twice as much time with them, and
half as much money.

—ABIGAIL VAN BUREN

I sat at the kitchen table of a new friend's home, deep in conversation as my two children played with some of her eleven. Yes, eleven. Between sips of hot lentil soup and side glances to make sure my baby, Elena, wasn't covering their expansive book collection in teeth marks, the topic of laundry came up. I felt an immediate flood of tension. *She barely knows me, and now I might disclose our unspeakable kids' clothes situation.*

Kids' stuff was a real source of reactivity for me before my decluttering journey began. Just that morning I had angrily stuffed fistfuls of kids' clothes in the trash can so I wouldn't have to wash and fold them again. A few days ago, I had chucked a toy across the room, embedding it snugly between the couch cushions. At times I'd think of Paul's words in Romans 7:15: "I do not understand what I do." When it came to my reactivity, they resonated.

My eyes shifted to the softly falling snow outside. I decided to be open. What did I have to lose? With her being a mother of eleven kids, I figured she could sympathize with laundry talk.

I took a deep breath. "I've been behind on laundry since our second baby was born a year ago," I confessed. "It's mainly kids' clothes. Washing them is no problem, but it's the folding and putting away part I can't seem to do. Honestly, since we still co-sleep, we just throw the clean laundry in the crib and dig it out of there."

She remained silent. Surely I had a "laundry chaos cohort" in this new friend. Surely, she had five stories that would each one-up my dig-from-the-crib system. But what she said surprised me. "Figure out a system now," she began gently. "The sooner the better."

While her response certainly wasn't the one I expected, it was the one I needed. *Figure out a system.* I felt something shift within. I was being firmly challenged to step out of the overwhelm. Maybe a clutter-free home with kids wasn't unattainable. Maybe I could declutter my kids' stuff—toys, clothes, all of it—and finally counter the chaos that accompanied their copious stuff piles. All I had to do was figure out how.

Decluttering Kids' Clothes

The solution came while packing for our annual Thanksgiving trip outside Seattle: What if the only clothes I had to manage for my two children were the week's worth of outfits that I had packed into this neatly ordered suitcase? Rolling clothes tightly, I fit five outfits per child in the suitcase. If I could do laundry as needed, this amount should be sufficient. I decided that if our girls thrived with limited outfits on this vacation, then I'd replicate this "suitcase experiment" at home.

As expected, fewer outfits led to content, adequately clad children—and *a lot* less laundry to do.

When I got home, I hauled the carry-on into their room and surveyed the disorder of their overstuffed closets. "They don't need or use all this stuff—the multiple matching pajamas, the rows of colorful dresses, the drawers teeming with T-shirts. They didn't miss it on vacation and won't now," I thought.

For the first time in a long time, I felt a spark of excitement while staring at piles of clothes.

Motivated to re-create the suitcase experiment, I lined up a good chunk of childcare and got to work. First, I grabbed our suitcase and, imagining a week's vacation, packed only what our girls needed. I zipped the suitcase and set it aside. I pulled the rest of the clothes off hangers and out of drawers and put them in bags to save or donate.

Hours later I had three big bags of kids' clothes ready to donate and one bag to save for next season. Then I opened the suitcase.

Organizing was easy. When tightly rolled, my daughters' wardrobe items all fit neatly into their own ten-by-twenty-inch drawer: a row for dresses, a row for pants, a row for long-sleeved shirts, and a corner for underwear. A few special dresses hung in the closet. Every item had a home, and every item was something my daughters frequently wore.

If you have kids, you too can re-create the suitcase experiment. Here's how:

STEP 1. Get a large suitcase (or multiple suitcases if you have a large family). Imagine you're going on a week-long vacation where you can do laundry as needed.

STEP 2. Pack a week's worth of clothes for each of your children (include them in the decluttering process if you feel they are ready to help—more on this in the "Kid-Related FAQs" section). Consider weekly activities (swimming, soccer) and favorite outfits. Experiment with keeping fewer outfits than you think you'll need.

STEP 3. Separate the remaining clothes into donate and keep piles, and bag each pile separately. Put them out of sight for a while and see if your children miss anything. You can easily retrieve an item if they request it. Your "keep" bag is for out-of-season clothing (I kept five to six out-of-season outfits per child).

STEP 4. Unpack the suitcase and find a home for each item. This is where it will go when you put away laundry or quickly tidy up a room.

STEP 5. Tweak the process as needed. Remember, this is an experiment. You can make changes until you have a system that works best for your family. (Read about our laundry system in chapter 14.)

Kids' Capsule Wardrobe

If you're wanting to create a capsule wardrobe for your kids, you may consider making a master list of all the clothing your child will need for all seasons.

This will give you guidelines on how many total clothing items to keep. Here are the lists we used for our children:

The master list for our girls included:

6 shirts (3 long-sleeved, 3 short-sleeved)
6 dresses (3 longed-sleeved, 3 short-sleeved)
4 pairs of pants (3 leggings, 1 pair of jeans)
3 pairs of shorts
2 pairs of pajamas (one for summer, one for winter)
1 swimsuit
Sneakers
Flip flops
Dress shoes
8 pairs of underwear
6 pairs of socks
Cardigan
Lightweight jacket

The master list for our boy included:

10 shirts (5 short sleeved, 5 long sleeved)
1 pair of jeans
3 pairs knit pants
3 pairs of shorts
2 pairs of pajamas (one for summer, one for winter)
1 swimsuit
Sneakers
Waterproof sandals
Dress shoes
8 pairs of underwear

6 pairs of socks

Lightweight jacket

For more on creating a capsule wardrobe for kids, go to www.richinwhatmatters.com and search "capsule."

My sign that the suitcase experiment was an immediate success was the day I caught Eva putting her clothes away independently. She had gone from toting piles of clothes around the house like it was a game to voluntarily caring for her clothes, all because of an environment change.

The logical next step seemed to be decluttering kids' toys.

Decluttering Kids' Toys

Today, children in the US make up 3.1 percent of the world's kid population, but US families buy more than 40 percent of the toys purchased globally.[1] In her book *Born to Buy*, sociologist Juliet Schor reports that the average American child receives seventy new toys a year.[2]

But studies show that children who own fewer toys are far from deprived. An environment with fewer toys fosters deeper, more meaningful, more creative play and teaches children to be more than consumers.

Lisa M. Ross, in a book with Kim John Payne, *Simplicity Parenting: Using the Extraordinary Power of Less to Raise Calmer, Happier, and More Secure Kids*, outlines the problem of rampant toy consumption:

Carl Jung said that children do not distinguish between ritual and reality. In the world of childhood, toys are ritual objects with powerful meaning and resonance. To a child, a mountain of toys is more than something to trip over. It's a topographical map of their emerging worldview. The mountain, casting a large symbolic shadow, means "I can choose this toy, or that, or this one way down here, or that: They are all mine! But there are so many that none of them have value. I must want something else!" This worldview shapes their emotional landscape as well; children given so very many choices learn to undervalue them all, and hold out—always—for whatever elusive thing isn't offered. "More!"[3]

A continual stream of stuff begets a desire for even more. Often, parents are the source of the toy infestation in their homes. In feeding children's desire for the newer and bigger, we're raising children primed for a lifetime of material consumption. The good news? It's not too late to change this pattern.

Five Steps to Declutter Kids' Toys

STEP 1. If you can, line up childcare for your children, preferably out of the house. Payne recommends doing this initial toy purge without your child, regardless of their age, so they don't "profess undying love for all of the things they never play with, the toys that have been broken and long forgotten."[4] Then collect all the toys in the home into one room, even if it's a staggering amount.

STEP 2. Designate one eighteen-gallon storage tote for toys you will keep. Then, braving the possibly-mammoth toy mound, separate the toys into three piles: beloved toys that are played with daily, toys that serve a purpose for imaginary play (also known as open-ended toys, which are toys that can be played with multiple ways, like dress-up clothes and magnetic tiles), and toys that aren't played with daily. I recommend keeping only toys in the first two categories.

STEP 3. Place all beloved toys and open-ended toys in the eighteen-gallon tote. Then fill heavy-duty blackout trash bags with the rest. Scoop up armfuls of unloved stuff and dump it into the dark abyss. Remind yourself that, ultimately, this is for your children's good and for the good of your entire family—because it is. When I did this, 10 percent of our toys remained.

STEP 4. Next, put the trash bags out of sight. Don't donate anything yet. Once the environment is reset, you will want to watch how your kids respond. This observation phase will allow your children to ask for an out-of-sight toy if they remember it and want it.

STEP 5. Finally, withdraw about ten toys from the "favorites tote" and organize them in the areas where your children play, leaving a small number of beloved toys visible.

The Box-and-Rotate System

When you set loving limits on the number of toys in the home or the amount of space toys can take up, you may feel like the "bad guy" at first, but you are helping your children in two ways. Setting clear, consistent limits helps children feel more secure and prepares them for adulthood. (Boundaries prevent them from developing a sense of entitlement.) And research indicates that having fewer toys "invites deeper play and engagement. An avalanche of toys invites emotional disconnect and a sense of overwhelm."[5]

After three months, you will have a feel for what your children play with and what they don't. Now is the time to start donating, or "rehoming," toys that are no longer played with.

Next, set up a toy rotation system. Every couple of weeks, rotate five to ten "new" toys from storage into the home, placing the recently-played-with toys back into the tote in storage. Here's a simple rule to know if too many toys have rotated into your home: If it takes your kids more than five minutes to tidy their toys independently, then you likely have too many toys out.

Consider setting up a routine where before Christmas and birthdays the toy tote is decluttered. Help your children choose what they'd like to let go of to make room for anything new they receive.

While owning fewer toys sounds countercultural—and it is—your kids will realize that happiness doesn't come from material wealth. You can still spoil your kids, but spoil them with quality time, attention, and experiences, not stuff.

Kid-Related FAQs

Should I involve my child in decluttering their stuff?

Yes, absolutely. Many cultures peg age seven as the age of reason. Around age seven, children have the cognitive flexibility to understand that the world is not all about them. This is prime time to let your kiddos make decisions about their stuff. You know your child best and can choose whether you involve them in the initial toy purge or only maintenance decluttering.

Regardless of your choice, start the "we don't need to keep it all" conversations early. A three-year-old can learn simple boundaries around toys, like all his toys needing to fit in one basket; when the basket is full, then old toys go to a new home. Or when a new toy comes into his life, an old one goes out of his life.

What if my kids won't let go of their stuff?

Often when you're talking to children, what matters isn't *what* you say but *how* you say it. If you're talking about letting go of toys but you're afraid this could harm or upset your child, they will sense that. Work through your own hesitations before talking to your children so you can do it from a place of assurance and calm. Family meetings are a great place to have these types of discussions and to set new boundaries as a team.

In my experience, playing the role of "decluttering dictator" is futile. Instead, give your child ownership of the decluttering project. This could be as simple as walking into your child's room with a reusable shopping bag and saying, "We've been very blessed to have everything we need. Many kids don't. Some kids don't even have toys. Here's a bag for you. If you see something in your room you don't need anymore, feel free to put it in the bag. Next week I'll be taking a load of stuff to help out these children. If you have anything you want to add, I can take it too." Then smile and leave the room. Let go of your expectations and observe what happens. If your child doesn't respond the first time, try again in a week or two.

Most children are naturally generous and, when given ownership, will likely respond.

How do I declutter kids' artwork?

Involve your children in the keep-or-toss decision-making process as soon as their art session is finished or when they bring new artwork into your home. Consistently asking your child whether the artwork is "ta da" or "ta dump" plants the seed that not everything needs to be kept. Admire their art, commenting matter-of-factly on several features of it. ("You used green on the girl's dress.") Then ask your children to help you decide which pieces to keep. ("Let's keep the most special ones! Which ones are those?") Recycle any unwanted art pieces immediately; display one to two favorites.

Artwork that is not recycled or displayed goes directly into our paper basket in a low kitchen cabinet. I tell our kids the artwork will stay in the "special paper place." Once the paper bin is full, revisit the artwork with your children, telling them, "The basket is full now, so we get to choose your very favorites to keep."

Very favorite artwork now goes into a portfolio. We use a three-ring binder with plastic page protectors. Our children each have a binder that stays in the book basket in their room. When the binder is full, the child gets to choose what to let go of to make room for new artwork. If your child makes frequent 3D art or creates art on extra-large paper, I'd suggest having a designated display place for this type of art. As new 3D or extra-large pieces come in, they can replace the ones on display. Store those that are no longer favorites out of sight, revisit them in several months' time, photograph them, and then give them away.

Consider repurposing any artwork that isn't deemed a
favorite. Use it as wrapping paper. Mail it to a grandparent,
aunt, uncle, or cousin. Take a photo of it so the child can
still see it anytime. (Let the child be the photographer—our
kids love to do this.) For more on decluttering kids' artwork,
visit www.richinwhatmatters.com and search "art."

What do I do about gift-giving?

Minimalist living isn't opposed to gift-giving; it's just focused
on gifting experiences instead of stuff. But even after you've
announced your minimalist manifesto to extended family,
loved ones may still want to give you and your kids more stuff.
Why? They want to show their love. Here's the good news:
They can still show their love without adding to your stuff.

You'll need to have a conversation with your loved ones
about gift-giving. The formula I've found most effective looks
like this: Be grateful + state your *why* + tell people what you'd
like them to do (instead of what you *don't* want them to do).
Here are some examples of what you could say:

We are blessed that you want to buy our girls gifts. With
two kids now, we'd love a family zoo pass. They'd love
this gift so much!

Or

We are so grateful that you want to give our children
many wonderful gifts. Our girls are really into baking
right now. They'd absolutely love new ingredients!

Ultimately, you can't control what people will purchase. But you can control your outlook and decide to be grateful. You also control what you decide to keep in your home after it has been given. The purpose of a gift is to show love. Once a gift is opened and the love behind it has been appreciated, the gift has served its purpose.

For more tips on navigating gift-giving, go to www.richinwhatmatters.com and search "gifts."

The Happy Box

I spent weeks decluttering my kids' stuff. Finally, the calm environment gave me space to observe my behavior. Culling kid-related clutter had greatly reduced my impatience, but it still arose at times. Within a week, I'd pinpointed a common cause of my reactivity—it flared most when I needed a break but hadn't taken one.

Author Viktor E. Frankl is attributed with saying, "Between stimulus and response there is a space. In that space is our power to choose our response. In our response lies our growth and our freedom."[6]

The antidote to reactivity is putting enough space between stimulus and response.

Reactivity activates the primitive part of the brain responsible for producing strong emotions like anger or fear. This cuts off our "thinking brain" and makes it hard for us to express spiritual fruits like patience and gentleness. Yet Paul tells us in his letter to the Philippians to "let your gentleness be evident to all" (4:5). To stay "gentle like Jesus," to respond and not react, is a game of nervous-system regulation and self-observation. Your job? To feel and observe your body tensing and insert a breath or break before acting impulsively.

To combat my lingering reactivity, I consulted my brain-guru therapist friend and, within days, had designed a toolbox called a "happy box." My happy box was a small box containing items that research has shown to change brain chemistry. The box's contents are meant to activate the senses and the vagus nerve, which calm the brain and nervous system respectively. My goal: to reset my mind in turbulent moments and reconnect with God.

Examples of Items in a "Happy Box"

- Sight: photos of happy moments, a liquid motion timer, a glitter jar
- Smell: essential oils in a roller bottle or small spray bottle (we use bergamot oil; studies show it calms the part of the brain that engages in overthinking), rose water, smelly markers
- Taste: small candies or peppermints, flavored lip balm
- Touch: a smooth rock (this can be placed on the neck if cold to stimulate the vagus nerve and promote relaxation and grounding[7]), silly putty, gel shapes, lotion
- Hearing: a small music box, a calming recorded message
- My box also contains colored pencils and paper. Coloring activates the frontal lobe, which means your brain is problem-solving again.[8]

I began taking "happy box breaks" by retreating briefly to my room when feeling overstimulated. I stopped pushing through tense moments, instead making space to determine my body and mind's underlying needs. If I couldn't leave the room, I brought the box to me. And if I couldn't access the box, I sang, hummed, or pretended to gargle (yes, this works) to stimulate the vagus nerve and reset.[9]

Soon Eva, always watching, followed suit, taking her own "happy box breaks" when needed or singing to support her tiny system when stressed. She was learning to take care of herself—to navigate her big feelings instead of running from them.

Our emotions are a gift from God. They give us information about our needs and where God wants to meet us in our lives. Whatever we are feeling is normal, valid, and good. Happy boxes help us return to a state of mind where we can connect with God, talk to him about our emotions, and truly process them, not avoid them.

Owning significantly less kids' stuff and having a tool to conquer reactivity will make your home and your mind calm. You can regain patience and refocus on God. Perhaps you'll feel like Jacob in Genesis 28:16, reawakening to God's presence by saying, "Surely the LORD is in this place, and I was not aware of it." He has always been there, and he is, and always will be, enough.

---

10 Kids' Items to Declutter

1. Toys your kids don't like or have outgrown
2. Broken toys
3. Multiples of anything

4. Toys you like and wish your kids played with but don't
5. Coloring books that have been completely colored through
6. Old school papers
7. Artwork that isn't your kids' very favorite
8. Clothes your kids have outgrown or no longer wear
9. Clothes received as gifts or hand-me-downs that aren't loved
10. Clothes that are beyond repair

Inner Decluttering Tool: Create Your "Happy Box"

Create a "happy box" for yourself and each of your children (let them help you make theirs). Model using the box to ground yourself and reset your nervous system anytime you're flooded with big feelings. Once calm, ask the Holy Spirit for an outpouring of patience and gentleness. Remind yourself that no one and no "things" have permission to hijack your nervous system. Remember: Calm, peace, and relaxation create a greater openness to God.

Outer Decluttering Tool: Dive into Decluttering Kids' Stuff

Decide which category of kids' stuff stresses you out most:

- Kids' clothes
- Kids' toys
- Kids' artwork

Choose one to declutter with the steps set out in the chapter. Kim John Payne says, "As you decrease the quantity of your child's toys and clutter, you increase their attention and their capacity for deep play."[10] By decluttering kids' stuff, by saying yes to simplifying, you are saying no to entitlement and overwhelm. Ultimately, you are giving your children a more meaningful childhood.

12

DECLUTTERING SENTIMENTAL ITEMS AND LETTING GO OF FEAR

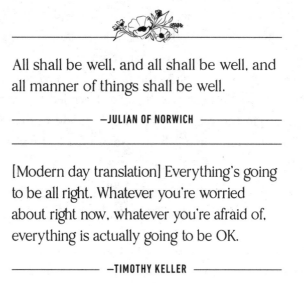

All shall be well, and all shall be well, and all manner of things shall be well.

————— —JULIAN OF NORWICH —————

[Modern day translation] Everything's going to be all right. Whatever you're worried about right now, whatever you're afraid of, everything is actually going to be OK.

————————— —TIMOTHY KELLER —————

One slow Saturday morning, I stood in our upstairs room, immersed in a quagmire of sentimental boxes I intended to declutter.

What would it feel like to surround myself only with things that supported the person God was calling me to become today, now? I pondered the question with the gravitas it deserved. Multiple descriptors arose: freeing, expansive, yet potentially dolesome, terrifying. To live fully for today would take a degree of trust I desired but wasn't sure I possessed. I scanned the sea of boxes and imagined myself slowly sinking, and Jesus gently coaxing, "You of little faith, why are you so afraid?" (Matthew 8:26).

Why *was* I so afraid? What about my past was more important than focusing on God and the present moment?

In Scripture, there are 365 instances of God telling his people to "fear not."[1] "Be not afraid" was frequently on Jesus's lips. Yet here I was, still afraid.

I started to cry as I stood there immobilized among the boxes—tears coming not at the idea of loss but at the realization of what I'd been withholding. I needed to trust God. Everything in those boxes was from him and ultimately his, but I was afraid to relinquish the trinkets that defined my past.

Why Sentimental Items Can Be Hard to Part With

If there's a category of your home that decluttering experts say to do last once you've fully developed your decluttering muscles, it's the sentimental items. The memories and emotions attached to sentimental items make them hard to declutter— even though they often have no real use or monetary value.[2]

Your attachments to these items may run so deep that you equate the possession with a person, an era, a place, or a feeling. The tiny first pair of shoes you bought your son on a whim represents early motherhood. The stuffed animal you snuggled nightly when you were seven embodies your childhood. The pair of paperweight ducks you used to play with at your grandmother's and inherited after her passing revive wonderful memories of her. To anyone else, these items could be considered junk, but to you, they are viscerally connected to who you are. Parting with them can feel painful—you fear losing an important part of your past and the associated memories.

But here's the truth: truly precious memories never dissipate, even when you discard the possessions associated with them. While I'm not recommending getting rid of every sentimental item, holding on to too many past objects can keep you from living fully in the present.

"It's not our memories but the person we have become because of those past experiences that we should treasure," Marie Kondo said. "This is the lesson that these keepsakes teach us when we sort them. By handling each sentimental item and deciding what to discard, you process your past."[3]

We live in the present moment—the place God waits to meet us. No matter how wonderful things were in the past, we cannot live there. Our possessions and living spaces should support the person we are becoming now, not the person we used to be.

Just because items were important to you at a certain point in life doesn't mean they hold value as you move into the next stage of life. If you're an empty nester holding on to baby items that you needed as a new parent, those items likely aren't useful now. You don't need a box full of onesies anymore. Keep your favorite and pass the rest on. If you're a mother in your forties, let go of the high school yearbooks that you treasured when you were eighteen (or rip out your favorite pages). If you're now married, release the journals you crafted when you were single. If five years ago was an intense time of grieving, let go of the boxes of letters that supported you during that time and select a couple to keep.

Letting go of emotion-laden items from past stages of life frees us to enter the present moment more fully. Letting go of sentimental items that feel like a part of you won't erase memories or change who you are, but instead will make space for you to grow into who God's calling you to become.

Decluttering Sentimental Items

Go through your sentimental items however you see fit—box by box, shelf by shelf—and be sure to hold every item while decluttering it. Use the tips below to help you let go of sentimental possessions.

Use the Spontaneous Combustion Question

The Minimalists recommend using the spontaneous combustion question to declutter sentimental items. Take a sentimental item in your hand and ask yourself, "How would I feel if this item spontaneously combusted?"[4]

Would you feel relieved? Then let that item go. Would you feel good, but a little guilty? Then take a picture of the item and then let it go. Would you feel devastated? Then that's an item you definitely want to keep.

If imagining your possession spontaneously combusting didn't do the trick, try asking this question: "Is this item holding me in the past, or freeing me to live in the present?" Any item that triggers guilt (the boxes of thirty-year-old musty baby clothes your mother-in-law dropped off for your new baby) or sadness (a deceased relative's living room set that you surprisingly inherited) is not freeing you to live fully in the present. While an item may seem to hold meaning or value, if it's anchoring you in the past, the cost of owning it is too "expensive."

Go Digital

Sentimental items may bring up good memories, but remember, your memories are within you, not within your stuff. Letting go of the item doesn't mean relinquishing the attached memory. To preserve the memory, could you take a picture of the item, create a "sentimental items" photo folder, and flip through it when desired? Same emotions, a lot less stuff.

Eliminate Duplicate Items

When decluttering, look for duplicate items that evoke similar memories. If you have thirteen souvenirs from your trip to Paris twenty years ago, could you keep just one? Hold on to the tiny-baker-man-with-a-beret-and-baguette magnet, display it proudly, and then photograph and let go of everything else.

Set Limits

You'll want to set limits when decluttering sentimental items. You may keep as many items as you choose, but fit them in one designated box (instead of fifteen). Plan to use the items you deem keep-worthy. I have one basket of sentimental items that I keep on the top shelf of my closet. I routinely pull down the basket, enjoy looking through the items, and often use them to tell stories about my life to our children. They can read my favorite card my grandmother wrote me, studying her slanted handwriting as they ask me about her life. They can fold their hands around the small wooden camel I purchased at an Egyptian market along the Nile. Holding the items helps make the stories come to life.

If these sentimental items were hidden throughout a spread of boxes in our upstairs room like they used to be, there'd be no enjoying them. I even have a sentimental item display spot in my closet where I put an item I'd like to see daily. I rotate this item from the basket, which helps me enjoy and use the items I've chosen to keep.

Streamline Your Photos

Sort your photographs into three piles: Love, Kind of love, and Don't love. Then keep only the ones you love. You likely won't miss the others. The work is tedious, but it's worth it if you plan to keep and enjoy photographs. Also consider using the spontaneous combustion question mentioned previously.

It's normal to feel like you're pitching memories; you're afraid they will become unretrievable. Try to reframe your thoughts this way: Instead of focusing on the photos you're releasing, think, "I am keeping my best memories." Trust your memory to God. Let him touch it and make it remember what he considers important. When you give him control, it's much easier to loosen your grip.

Choose a Photo Display

Next, choose how you want to display your favorite photos. I found traditional albums to be bulky and cumbersome, so I opted for four-by-six-inch albums that hold forty-eight photos each. I labeled the front cover of each album by category: trip to Europe, Eva's baby photos, Justin and Julia, childhood photos. Then I used one basket to hold the albums. The mini photo books provided a boundary for the number of photos I'd keep in each category, and the basket limited the number of albums I'd keep. I bring down the basket often for our kids so they can each grab a mini book and enjoy the photos.

If you want your photos out of sight, consider scanning them onto your computer. If you have a lot of pictures, I recommend outsourcing this task to a service like PhotoPanda. (If you send them a box of photos, they send you back a full flash drive.) Or consider using a digital picture frame to display photos in a clutter-free way.

Remember Your Family's Inheritance

One hard truth about our clutter is that, eventually, someone will have to decide what to do with every one of your possessions. Make decisions about your stuff now so others won't have to be overwhelmed by it later. Consider storing your treasures in a memorabilia bin that's been ruthlessly edited. The less you keep, the more meaningful your things become. In the words of author Patrick Lencioni, "If everything is important, then nothing is."[5]

If you're keeping mementos from your kids' childhood, here's another hard truth: They likely won't want them. That hospital bracelet, favorite baby spoon, adorable kindergarten assignment—they're all being saved . . . for *you*. Confidently let go of most childhood memorabilia knowing that, more than likely, your children won't want to inherit them. (Help your children design their own memorabilia bins too.)

By being intentional about the sentimental items you keep now, you lighten your family's load in the future.

Overcoming Fear

Letting go is an exercise in trust that has a ripple effect in other areas of your life. Every fearful situation you overcome rewires your brain pathways, methodically modifying your thinking. You *can* do it, and now you have proof. Letting go of hard-to-part-with items can even lead to letting go of a dead-end job, relinquishing unhealthy relationships, and jettisoning habits holding you back from your dreams and your God-given purpose.

When uprooting fear, the underlying question is, Whom or what do you trust? If your security is rooted in your belongings, then it's likely not in Jesus. In *Searching for and Maintaining Peace*, Jacques Philippe writes, "Our great drama is this: Man does not have confidence in God."[6]

While healthy fear keeps us from doing things we might regret, fear from the Enemy paralyzes us, keeps us from living out our dreams, and leads to mediocre lives.

Sometimes overcoming fear involves working with a therapist to archive emotions from past events that are still alive in our brains and controlling our behavior. Other times, it takes teasing out the fear-based beliefs or behaviors that persist simply because they were modeled for us at an impressionable age. (For example, maybe your parents projected a scarcity mindset.)

While these steps are helpful and often necessary to overcome fear, full healing includes a spiritual component: reestablishing Jesus as our source of security and trust. It requires letting go and letting God.

Philippe writes, "We cannot experience this support from God unless we leave Him the necessary space in which He can express Himself. I would like to make a comparison. As long as a person who must jump with a parachute does not jump out into the void, he cannot feel that the cords of the parachute will support him, because the parachute has not yet had the chance to open. One must first jump and it is only later that one feels carried."[7]

We humans are most fearful of the unknown. Yet God wants us to venture into the space "where feet may fail"[8] so that he can carry us. Maybe your unknown area is letting go of a basement full of stuff-filled boxes you know you're called to relinquish. Maybe it's saying yes to trying public speaking, adding a baby to your family, or starting a business. If God is calling you to it, trust that if you jump, you will feel carried.

The antidote to fear is trust.

Now when I catch myself entertaining fear, I ask myself one question: "What if everything works out?"

Read that again. *What if everything works out?*

He is within us. And he is for us. I choose to trust that it will.

---

10 Sentimental Items to Declutter

1. Photos that aren't your very favorites
2. Unloved yearbooks
3. Baby clothes (keep a couple of favorites per child)
4. Family heirlooms you're keeping because you think you "should"
5. Random travel souvenirs
6. Gifts you're keeping out of obligation

---

7. Random trinkets and "treasures"
8. Old T-shirts from memorable events
9. Journals from past seasons of life
10. Birthday cards or letters (keep one to two favorites per sender)

Inner Decluttering Tool: Anchor Your Mind in Trust

Psalm 16:8 says that by keeping our "eyes always on the LORD," we "will not be shaken."

Overcoming fear requires shifting our gaze toward God in prayer. Through prayer, we "taste and see how good the LORD is" (Psalm 34:8 CEB) and our minds begin to understand that he will sustain us even in the unknown.

Grab a pen and paper and write down four to five times in your life when you took a leap of faith, acting even when you didn't know how things would turn out. Now write the positive aspects that came from each action. Put this list next to your bed. Every night, make this list the last thing you read before sleeping. Conclude with a prayer: (Breathe in) "Jesus, (Breathe out) I trust you."

Now practice doing one out-of-the-norm thing this week that takes reliance on God.

- Invite a neighbor over for dinner, even though you don't know them well and aren't sure how it will go.
- Call a loved one you don't talk to often and tell them

you're thinking of them, even though it may feel uncomfortable.

- Start a conversation with a stranger while waiting in line, even though you're not sure how they will respond.
- Donate a hard-to-part-with item, even though it may feel unnatural.

Let Jesus carry you and he will.

Outer Decluttering Tool: Address the Sentimental Stuff

What would it feel like to surround yourself only with things that support the person you are becoming now, not the person you used to be? Journal your answer; use bullet points if that helps. Use your response as motivation to declutter.

Now commit to decluttering sentimental items using the practical tools mentioned in this chapter. Start with one of these steps:

- Set up a system for photos.
- Create a memorabilia box.
- Begin opening boxes of sentimental items, holding each one, and using the spontaneous combustion question to ruthlessly declutter them.

Trust that in letting go of old sentimental items, you are unearthing a better, more present life.

13

DECLUTTERING YOUR DIGITAL WORLD AND LETTING GO OF DISTRACTION

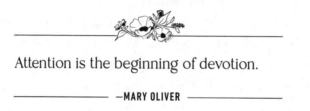

Attention is the beginning of devotion.

—MARY OLIVER

In *Hands Free Mama*, Rachel Macy Stafford writes about the "Disease of Distraction." Stafford says,

If you live in the twenty-first century,
Then you may be affected by this disease.
If you find yourself reaching for your phone instead of talking or playing with your kids,
If your calendar is filled with a constant flurry of activity,
If you feel like you never slow down,
If you get through the day and realize you haven't made eye contact or real conversation with someone you love,

Then you may be affected by the disease. . . .

If you constantly feel your attention being averted from what really matters to the insignificant and meaningless details of your life, then you might be familiar with The Disease of Distraction.[1]

During my decluttering journey, I discovered that I, like many people, suffered from the disease. I had slowed down considerably, ruthlessly uncluttered my calendar, and redirected much of my life toward what mattered. I tried to convince myself I was symptom free. But in the quiet moments, an interior nagging carried a different message.

God confirmed this on an evening walk when I noticed that I was staring at my cell phone, eyes hypnotized by the soft glow of the screen. A soft, clear voice stopped me mid-scroll: *"How can I connect with you when you're so often like that?"* My feet froze. His tone sounded gentle, almost sad.

What had started out as blogging led to a growing social media presence, which then led to an unchecked compulsion to "research this for an article" or to check Instagram to view comments and likes. By now I had a two-minute "phone twitch loop": check texts, then email, then Facebook, Instagram, and blog hits—all in one fell swoop that I ran multiple times an hour.

Simply laying eyes on that shiny, light pink phone case was enough to propel me to engage. I was alarmed by the velocity at which I could go into my phone twitch loop. One minute I'd be cooking dinner, conversing with my daughter; the next minute I'd catch myself midway through my loop, about to respond to a Facebook comment, wondering, "Why am I on Facebook now and, more importantly, why is this so hard to put down?" That six-inch rectangle had the upper hand on my actions simply by being within eyesight.

As I walked and thought, I realized my phone habits were thieving moments of my one life by shifting my eyes away from what and who really mattered. I couldn't truly see what I was missing until I looked up. I knew that with my eyes continually locked on a screen, I was missing the details of my life. I was missing connection with God.

That weekend, I sought out a mentor from our church. He listened diligently as I described the disease of distraction and my most recent symptom: compulsive phone checking. His response, although annoyingly Socratic, was what I needed to hear. He simply asked me to consider the symbol on the back of my iPhone: an apple with a bite out of it.

To a Christian, it might as well be the symbol for temptation. He spoke of freedom and my ability to control my actions and choose the good. If I felt the need to grab my phone whenever I saw it, was I truly free? Who controlled whom?

I am certainly not alone in struggling with digital addiction. We are a society attached to our devices. Consider these recent statistics from ConsumerAffairs:

- Americans look at their phones 144 times a day.
- Americans spend an average of 4 hours and 30 minutes a day on their phone (over 2 of those hours are spent on social media).
- Nearly 57 percent of Americans consider themselves "mobile phone addicts."
- Three in four Americans admit to feeling uncomfortable without their phones.

- About 25 percent of children have their first phone at 10.7 years old, while 75 percent have one by 12.6 years old.[2]

Lack of autonomy around our phones restricts us from living life on purpose. And herein lies the problem. Cal Newport, author of *Digital Minimalism*, says, "The urge to check Twitter or refresh Reddit becomes a nervous twitch that shatters uninterrupted time into shards too small to support the presence necessary for an intentional life."[3]

We weren't designed to live lives of constant interruption, focused more on the digital world than the physical and spiritual worlds around us. Smartphone use is changing our brain structure and function, reducing gray matter in a way that mirrors chemical addictions. "The smartphone is the modern-day hypodermic needle, delivering digital dopamine 24/7 for a wired generation," says Anna Lembke, author of *Dopamine Nation*.[4] Constant phone checking is facilitating addiction, raising our stress levels, absorbing our time, hijacking our focus, and causing us to miss out on our lives.[5]

Smartphone use, and especially social media use, is also impeding our brains' ability to deeply engage in spiritual practices like prayer. "Social media . . . trains people to think in ways that are exactly contrary to the world's wisdom traditions [including Christianity]," Jonathan Haidt says in *The Anxious Generation*. "Think about yourself first; be materialistic, judgmental, boastful, and petty; seek glory as quantified by likes and followers."[6]

Haidt explains that processing events from an egocentric point of view activates an area of the brain called the default mode network. This is the neural network that must be quiet—not activated—for us to "deeply connect to something beyond ourselves."[7]

Constant social media use is resulting in brain changes that lessen our ability to raise our minds to God. "To experience more self-transcendence," Haidt says, "we need to turn down the things in our lives that . . . bind us tightly to our egos, such as time on social media."[8]

What can we do about this? The first step is awareness. The second is practicing digital minimalism.

Newport defines digital minimalism as "a philosophy of technology use in which you focus your online time on a small number of carefully selected and optimized activities that strongly support things you value, and then happily miss out on everything else."[9]

---

10 Ways to Limit Distractions and Reclaim Your Time

1. **KEEP MORNINGS QUIET.** When you look at your phone first thing in the morning, you focus on what your phone says is most urgent, not what matters most to you. Try starting the day with quiet and stillness instead of screen time. Put your phone in airplane mode before you go to bed and keep it that way until you're ready to interact with it the next day.

2. **MAKE YOURSELF LESS AVAILABLE.** Let go of the idea that you have to be available to everyone all the time. You have no obligation to be constantly "on call." When responding immediately to dings becomes habitual, broken attention becomes your norm. Plus, if your phone frequently takes priority over

the person you're with, they may start questioning their importance to you.

3. **CONSOLIDATE TEXTING.** Instead of responding to text messages as they're received, consolidate your texting. First, keep your phone in Do Not Disturb mode by default (you can adjust the settings so calls from a selected list, like your Favorites, still come through). Texts will be seen only by opening up the app, making them like emails.

Next, schedule specific times for texting—consolidated sessions where you review and respond to previously received texts. You may choose to text back and forth for a few minutes, but then turn the phone back to Do Not Disturb mode and continue with your day. Despite making you less available, consolidated texting can strengthen your relationships, as your messages become more deliberate.

4. **RETHINK EMAIL.** Remove email notifications from your phone. Maybe even remove your email app entirely. The time it takes to download the app again will give you time to ask yourself questions. Do you *really* need to check your email again, or are you checking it out of habit? Behavior change requires putting space between a stimulus and a response. Remove what triggers you to refresh your email feed and you'll do it much less often.

Set specific times to check email, and then limit all email correspondence to those times. Maybe this means checking email at noon and again in the evening. Or maybe you dedicate a block of time several days a week to complete all email-related work.

If you're not ready to remove the email app from your phone, then consider adjusting your settings so that your email app only refreshes every hour.

5. **RAISE YOUR AWARENESS.** Behind social media apps are highly intelligent designers working to get you to spend as much time on their platforms as possible. Any app with a "like" button capitalizes on the fact that our brains release far more dopamine when our reward is unexpected than when it is predictable. (Psychology calls this "variable reinforcement.") These apps are like slot machines that leave us constantly wondering, "What will I get next?" Keep this in mind before you log on. Don't fall into their time-sucking traps.

6. **CHANGE HOW YOU USE SOCIAL MEDIA.** Reduce the temptation to mindlessly scroll by removing all social media apps from your phone. Begin using social media only on your laptop, and schedule a set amount of time for social media use. Maybe you check it for thirty minutes in the evening three times a week, or ten minutes a day after lunch. Prepare yourself to be amazed at how much more free time you have. (Remember, the average American spends over two hours a day on social media.)

If you're not ready to remove social media apps, at least remove all notifications from these apps. You can also set time limits on your social media usage in your phone's Settings or use apps like App-Block or FocusMe to lock yourself out of social media apps for set periods of time.

7. **ENGAGE IN HIGH-QUALITY LEISURE.** Use this extra time to engage in high-quality leisure activities. Learn a new skill (ukulele, knitting, a second language). Go on more walks. Join a cause you feel passionate about. High-quality leisure is essential to increased focus. Novelty enhances mood and motivation, while rest and play refuel our creativity and capacity to work.[10]

8. **SPEND TIME IN SILENCE.** Compulsive smartphone use is driven by an imbalance of two pathways in the brain: the "liking" system and the "wanting" system.[11] When the "wanting" system is in overdrive, we make choices that we don't rationally like. This is the case in chemical addictions and behavioral addictions alike.[12] Silence helps rebalance these two brain pathways, resulting in less compulsive phone use.

9. **INTENTIONALLY SPEND TIME ALONE.** Before cell phones, our days were full of moments ripe for solitude and self-reflection: waiting in line, walking down the street, cleaning the house, doing yard work, or taking the subway. Today, these are all opportunities to plug in. Challenge yourself not to use your phone during these natural breaks and instead spend time with your thoughts (or better yet, with God).

10. **CHALLENGE THE BELIEF THAT YOU ALWAYS NEED YOUR PHONE.** Simply seeing your phone can trigger the desire to use it, so intentionally keep your phone out of sight

more often. Leave your phone at home or in your car's glove compartment while running errands. Take walks without your phone or with your phone buried in the bottom of a backpack. Ask yourself, "Do I really need this?" before automatically bringing your phone along.

Newport said, "Humans are not wired to be constantly wired."[13] If you're as exhausted by your compulsive smartphone engagement as I was, I encourage you to try a couple of ideas from "10 Ways to Limit Distractions and Reclaim Your Time." Practicing digital minimalism allows our smartphones to work to our advantage, supporting our best life instead of distracting us from it. We only get one life. Let's not miss it because of an unchecked attachment to our screens.

Connection over Distraction

Even at the height of my awareness, I was still averaging almost four hours of screen time on my phone each day. I was sure the number of minutes a day I was truly available to God was far less. I struggled with guilt, shock, confusion.

When I wanted to escape a hard moment—like when my kids wanted my help but I was exhausted—I still sometimes instinctively reached for my phone and began to scroll. It felt better than listening to whining. But I had to ask myself, "Who is controlling whom?" I had to decide to put down my phone and go read a book with my toddler—to soak in the details of my life that I'd been missing.

Awareness continued to fuel my action. I put a rubber band around my phone to physically prevent me from unintentional scrolling. I bought an old-fashioned alarm clock, put my phone to bed in another room each night instead of letting it sleep within arm's reach, kept it on grayscale during the day, and began timing my daily social media with an alarm, stopping when it was time.

I also began answering texts in the evening once the girls were asleep, and I avoided my phone at all costs in the morning, giving that time to God. I prayed for the grace to stop checking it compulsively at red lights and took twenty-four-hour breaks from it each weekend (from noon Saturday to noon Sunday).

I knew if my phone-related choices continued unchecked, my distraction would cause me to overlook vital pieces of my one God-given life. As you consider your own digital decluttering journey, remember that the antidote to distraction is connection. It involves realizing that each moment of your life is fleeting, and vowing to enter deeply into those moments instead of throwing them away by unintentionally scrolling. In the words of author Mel Robbins, "Don't miss out on your life because you're too busy scrolling through someone else's."[14]

When you feel tempted to grab your phone, replace this twitch with some form of connection—reading a book with your child, holding an eye-to-eye conversation with your spouse, reading Scripture, or raising your mind to God.

Even when your inner and outer spaces are clutter free, if your digital practices still have the upper hand, your life will be anything but connected and meaningful.

Life is full of moments that only happen once in real time—moments we miss if our eyes are downward.

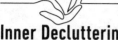

Inner Decluttering Tool: Replace Distraction with Connection

What times of day are you most tempted to entertain digital distractions? Some common times are first thing in the morning, the 3:00 p.m. slump, after dinner, and before bed. Catch yourself and replace the distraction with some form of connection instead: call a friend, write a letter, read a book to your child, invite a neighbor on a walk, talk to God. Simply raising your awareness by identifying your digital "red zones" will help you choose connection at this time instead of distraction.

Also, observe what you do during the natural breaks of your day (waiting in line, lunch break). Fight against using those times to scroll and use them to connect with God instead. (Use those times to ask him for the grace to use your phone with intention.)

Outer Decluttering Tool: Detach from Your Phone

Change your physical environment to make your phone less accessible, especially during times you're most tempted to engage in unintentional scrolling.

- Keep your phone out of the bedroom in the mornings and evenings.
- When driving, bury it in the bottom of a purse or somewhere out of reach.
- When home, have a designated place for it where you can hear it but not see it (mine is in the top of the hall closet).

Spend less time near your phone and you'll begin using it with increased intention.

14

MAINTENANCE DECLUTTERING

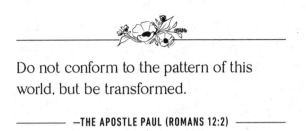

Do not conform to the pattern of this
world, but be transformed.

—THE APOSTLE PAUL (ROMANS 12:2)

Nine months after I embarked on my decluttering journey, I'd sifted through every clutter category. Every
physical thing in our home that wasn't my husband's had
been handled and then either retained or rehomed, culminat-
ing in the release of 75 percent of our possessions. The feel
and appearance of our home had been transformed. While it
still required some upkeep—it didn't clean itself—the time
commitment for upkeep was, well, minimal. My outer home
aligned, at long last, with my simplified vision for it, and I had
an abiding feeling that I'd found my life again under all that
stuff I'd cleared out.

But enmeshed in this "I'm living the dream" feeling, I for-
got whose dream it was. And under the influence of glossy
Pinterest posts and Instagram-worthy images, I began thinking

our home had to perpetually portray a polished image. I soon concluded that our home shouldn't be messy or have things out of place. But it turns out that making minimalism moral is a slippery slope.

One memorable Tuesday, I was tidying before a playdate—the first time anyone had entered our home since we'd officially finished decluttering. So naturally, I spent the entire hour before our guests arrived vacuuming, scrubbing baseboards, buffing fingerprints off the fridge, and essentially deep cleaning the entire home. I intermittently sweated profusely, barked at the kids, and finally resorted to giving them screen time so they didn't "mess anything up" before our guests arrived. (If you have or ever had a toddler, then you know.) The house looked great, but why didn't I feel at peace?

My friend walked through our front door and her eyes widened while I imagined she was processing internal before-and-after images. "Your home looks amazing," she finally breathed. I felt a momentary surge of pride and then a strong return of that I'm-not-really-at-peace feeling.

That evening, once our kids were asleep, I spent my last hour of the day talking with God. I told him the day had been exhausting. I told him *this* wasn't what I'd signed up for either. Had I come full circle? From the debilitating weight of clutter to an all-encompassing desire to maintain an image?

I grabbed *He and I* by Gabrielle Bossis, one of my all-time favorite spiritual reads, and immediately read, "Place me before each of your actions. What is your goal? Is it I? What is the object of your love?"[1]

The object of my love, that day, had still been stuff. While I hadn't been tempted to purchase shiny trinkets, I had tried to organize my remaining items in a perfect, Pinterest-approved fashion. But true order isn't about the way your house looks. It's about putting God before all things.

Although I no longer conformed to materialism, I had succumbed to the forces of Instagram influencers and Pinterest photos. So I pushed back. I allowed our uncluttered home to look more lived in instead of always tidy, knowing that messes often meant I'd chosen to play with my kids instead of cleaning up. I knew that with less stuff, it would take little time to reset an area when the moment was right.

You too can enjoy "messy minimalism," where the end goal isn't perfection. "Minimalism doesn't mean always tidy," writes author Rachelle Crawford. "It just means easily tidied."[2]

What does that look like in practice? It involves avoiding conformity and being overly influenced by others.

Transformed, Not Conformed

Our hearts and our homes alike require maintenance. Inner and outer decluttering is not a one-and-done effort. The process is ongoing. Once you've done the initial declutter, you'll need maintenance decluttering tools to ward off old habits or societal pressures that could cause you to regress.

For much of our lives, we are navigating various forces that cause us to either conform to the world or be transformed by Christ. Habits, thought patterns, daily rhythms, relationships, activities, and environments all affect our formation. Like it or not, we are all influenced. What we look at, whom we spend time with, and how we think all affect who we become.

We need awareness and planning (not to mention grace) to manage these forces. The goal is to develop habits, thought patterns, and daily rhythms that maintain an outer home that's free of physical clutter and an inner home with space for union with God.

The patterns of the world aren't going away. Advertisements continue to beckon, hurry is the new baseline speed, and distracting devices are rewiring our brains. Novelist Flannery O'Connor advised, "Push back against the age as hard as it pushes against you."[3]

In *Practicing the Way*, John Mark Comer writes that (inner and outer) transformation comes from taking up "a whole constellation of life choices that's different from the majority culture around us—to make choices that aim our love and longing at union with God and our formation into his likeness."[4]

If we want to resist worldly patterns like reactivity, hurry, and materialism, we need maintenance decluttering tools for our hearts and homes. Let's start with physical spaces.

Maintenance Mode

Maintaining a clutter-free home—not a perfect home—requires new habits. Clutter attracts clutter, so if you start leaving your receipts and car keys on the kitchen counter, soon a random assortment of pens, kids' artwork, and stray coins will follow. Everything in your home now has a "home"—you simply need to return it. In the words of Marie Kondo, author of *The Life-Changing Magic of Tidying Up*, "Clutter is caused by a failure to return things to where they belong."[5] In short, don't put it down; put it away.

Daily Maintenance Tasks

Two-Minute Tasks

David Allen's book *Getting Things Done* introduces the guideline that if a task takes less than two minutes to complete, you should do it now. Author Gretchen Rubin's one-minute rule follows the same principle. Doing the little tasks immediately and consistently leads to a tidier home. Here are one- to two-minute tasks to keep your home tidy. Plan to do these daily:

Make your bed.

Hang up your coat.

Place shoes in designated spots.

Put clothes away or in the hamper after wearing them.

Recycle junk mail.

Put away kitchen appliances after use (toaster, coffee maker).

File papers.

Pick up toys (teach your kids to do this).

Empty full trash cans.

Pick things up off the floor right away.

Put away bathroom toiletries after use.

Do whatever presents itself next, as long as it takes less than two minutes to complete.

When developing these daily two-minute tidying habits, post a note somewhere you'll see it often that reads "If it only takes two minutes, do it now!" Keeping this idea fresh in your mind increases the likelihood that you'll act accordingly. Momentum builds upon momentum.

For example, making your bed first thing in the morning sets the tone for your day. You'll carry this mindset into other parts of your day, increasing the probability that you'll take action. What starts with a made bed soon becomes clear kitchen countertops and floors without clothes piles.

Again, approach these tasks with flexibility and grace. God and the people in your home matter more than the home itself. Connect your tidying tasks to prayer by assigning a prayer intention to each one. If hanging up your clothes becomes a prayer for your friend, then your work has gone from monotonous to meaningful.

Over-Two-Minute Tasks

Several daily tasks take more than two minutes, such as unloading and reloading the dishwasher, resetting the main living area each evening, and, some days, washing and putting away laundry.

Speaking of laundry, here's our current system: We now do laundry almost daily. We no longer own a hamper or laundry basket. Dirty clothes—darks and lights—go straight into the washing machine, and we wash them when it's full. Then clean clothes get put away right away. I've found not owning a laundry basket encourages us to put laundry away daily. This task usually takes ten minutes.

Just because your space is clutter free doesn't mean your

new habits will be resistance free. On days when devoting even two minutes to a task seems hard, mindset hacks can help you take action.

CONSIDER THE SEVENTEEN-SECOND RULE

In his book *Pivot and Go*, mental skills specialist David Nurse outlines the seventeen-second rule.[6] When we're faced with a task, Nurse writes that seventeen seconds is all it takes for us to go from unenthused to engaged. Knowing that our mindset can shift once we simply start a task is essential for maintaining an uncluttered home.

Don't feel like putting away laundry even though it obviously needs to be done? Set a timer and get to work. Don't feel like putting away the dishes? All you have to get through is the first seventeen seconds of work for your resistance to fade. Soon you'll have the piles put away and be pleased with the clear space.

REALIZE HOW LONG TASKS TAKE

A daunting task can seem doable when you know how much time it will require. Go ahead and time yourself doing routine tasks in your home so you know how long they take. I've found this especially helpful when resetting our home at night. A glance across a disorderly room, especially when I'm tired, can make the task a bit overwhelming. Then I remind myself it takes only five minutes to retrieve throw pillows, fold a blanket, and return out-of-place items to their homes. Reframing the task in this way makes me feel like I have the upper hand. It gives me a you've-got-this mentality, which makes taking action easier.

Weekly Maintenance Tasks

One powerful weekly maintenance tool is a complete home reset. Designate a time to do this each week. I like to reset our home on Saturday afternoon, to prepare for a restful Sunday and a smoother week ahead. Teach your kids how to assist you with these tasks and how to do age-appropriate tasks independently.

Any items lingering in the laundry area need to be washed, dried, folded, and put away. (Use this time to notice what wardrobe items aren't even making it into the laundry. If no one is wearing them, you can likely let them go.) Bathrooms need weekly attention. (During this cleaning and reset, scan for empty product containers or other unused items and dispose of them.)

Walk through your living room, bedroom, and kids' rooms, returning any misplaced items to their homes. (Here again, scan for possessions that no longer serve you or your kids.)

Always keep a donate box or bag available, and add in unused or unloved items as they surface. I call ours the "What if we didn't own this?" bag. It's a reusable grocery bag that hangs in our hall closet. At the end of the month, if we haven't needed the items in the bag, then I deem them as clutter and let them go.

Consider using the "one in, one out" rule during your weekly home reset. As mentioned before, the premise of the rule is simple: For each new thing you bring into your home, one thing has to leave. If you acquired a new shirt that week, then choose one from your closet to donate. If your child got a new toy, then have him choose one to let go of.

Quarterly Maintenance Guidelines

The changing of the seasons is a great time to revisit clutter categories within your home. You can reuse the decluttering tools in this book to do a more in-depth maintenance declutter four times a year. If you prefer, you can also pair quarterly decluttering with New Year's, spring cleaning, back-to-school, and pre-holidays instead of the changing seasons. Choose your four maintenance decluttering sessions now and write them on your calendar.

During your quarterly declutter, spend time in the storage area of your home. Is there anything boxed away you've been meaning to let go of? Now is the time. If you're transitioning between seasonal wardrobes, let go of items you've outgrown or never wore. Reevaluate your kids' possessions. What have they outgrown? Did you just file taxes and have old papers you can now shred, digitize, or recycle? Are there any unloved holiday decorations it's time to let go of?

Even when we intend to be the tenacious gatekeeper of our home, things still enter our home that don't serve a purpose in our lives. We don't use them, love them, or need them. The purpose of material possessions is to be used for some good. If we're holding on to items that have no value or that we have simply outgrown, we are keeping them from potentially fulfilling their true purpose in someone else's life.

Change Your Buying Habits

Your solid maintenance routines and seamless home systems won't matter much if you haven't stopped the steady stream of material possessions coming into your home. Constantly adding in more stuff simply isn't conducive to a clutter-free home. In The Minimalists' book *Love People, Use Things*, Joshua Fields Millburn and Ryan Nicodemus outline six questions to ask yourself before making a purchase.[7] Remember, marketers are trained to beguile you so you'll buy. Consider these questions as your shield in the current battle for your brand loyalty and hard-earned cash.

---

6 Questions to Ask Before Making a Purchase

1. **AM I FEELING PRESSURED TO BUY THIS?** If you feel external pressure to make a purchase, pause and question why. Your worth and identity aren't found in your stuff. Buy it if it adds value to your life, not to impress anyone else. Millburn said, "The problem arises when we feel external pressure to acquire, as if new trinkets were a shortcut to a more complete life."[8]

2. **WILL THIS ADD VALUE TO MY LIFE?** Before purchasing an item, hold it in your hand (or if you're shopping online, imagine it in your hand) and consider its purpose. Be candid. Does the item have a specific function that no other item has? Does the item serve a specific aesthetic purpose? A home containing things that add value is a home that supports a more meaningful life.

3. **CAN I AFFORD IT?** Just because you can buy something doesn't mean you can afford it. The peace that comes with living debt free and within your means is worth more than anything you can buy.

4. **IS THIS THE BEST USE OF THIS MONEY?** Even if you can

---

afford something, it's worth asking if purchasing it is the best use of your money. Could the money serve you better if used for another purpose? Investing in retirement? Rent? A family vacation? If your money could be put to better use, Millburn asks, "Why not avoid the purchase and allocate the dollars to the most effective place?"[9]

5. **WHAT'S THE ACTUAL COST?** Everything we bring into our lives has a claim on some of our time, energy, and attention. Possessions must be cleaned, maintained, picked up, put away, and repaired. When we stop and consider the actual cost of an item, we realize it goes well beyond its price tag. Before buying something, add up *all* the costs. Choosing not to purchase the item might mean freeing up valuable resources to focus more on what truly matters.

6. **WOULD THE BEST VERSION OF ME BUY THIS?** If the best version of you wouldn't buy an item, then don't. Intuitively, most of us know whether a purchase is right, but we're good at justifying our spending. We coax ourselves into believing we *deserve* a possession or we *need* something to feel successful. Before making a purchase, pray for guidance and ask yourself if you really need to buy the item. Consider your gut feeling. If it's an uneasy one, listen and don't make the purchase.

Millburn said, "The easiest way to declutter your stuff is to avoid bringing it home in the first place."[10]

Consider experimenting with a shopping ban—a no-spend month (or three) where you buy nothing but consumables (such as groceries) and live with the durable goods (clothes, books, beauty products) you already own. Or consider a slow-buy month where you set a limit to what you buy that month (such as only two new items). These are powerful ways to break unhealthy shopping habits and free yourself to discover how little you need in order to be happy.

Inner Home Maintenance Decluttering

While outer maintenance decluttering comes from our own willingness to roll up our sleeves and get to work, inner home decluttering relies on a power beyond ourselves. The transformation Jesus offers isn't so much something we work for as something we commit to receiving. It's a daily process of renewal, of opening more space in our heart for God, that occurs in a piecemeal fashion. Spiritual growth is a practice, and it's ultimately God's work.

But we get to participate.

While on earth Jesus often uttered, "Come, follow me."[11] He wanted to gently encourage people to give his way of life a try. His invitation to emulate his day-to-day habits is still extended to us today. And it's the secret to warding off worldly conformity.

So what are some habits of Jesus worth emulating? There's no set list. But here are several: sabbath, solitude, prayer, fasting, reading Scripture, living in community, generosity, service, and witness.[12] Emulating the practices of Jesus allows us to *really* know Jesus, *really* know ourselves, and then mold our lives more closely to Christ's.

Patterning our lives after Jesus's life also keeps us from acting like cogs in a consumeristic machine and helps us fix our eyes on things above. Engaging with the world as he did helps maintain clutter-free inner homes. Restlessness, comparison, hurry, reactivity, fear, distraction—it's all minimized when, bit by bit, we're becoming more like the author of life.

In what ways does your life align with how Jesus lived when he was on earth? By studying his daily habits, we learn how to flourish as human beings. But the way of Christ is not about checking off a lengthy list showcasing everything we've done. Jesus never said, "Do more and I'll love you more."

It may be helpful to think, "Subtraction, not addition." Remember, less is more. In the words of John Mark Comer, "Focus on what you're not going to do, to build margin into the architecture of [your life]."[13]

Ask yourself, "What influences do I need to push back against to make space for Jesus's lighter way of life?" Social media, television, harmful relationships, spending patterns, unhealthy environments, recurring thoughts—which are sources of inner clutter for you? Which prevent you from becoming like Jesus? Change how you interact with them—or let go of them completely. Then slowly adopt his practices.

All Christian formation involves counterformation.[14] These practices allow us to push back, to be in the world but not of it. They create time and space for us to access the presence and the power of the Spirit and, in doing so, be transformed from the inside out.[15]

Choosing the practices of Jesus—not the patterns of this world—allows him to shape you into a loving person and allows you to fulfill your God-given purpose during your brief stint on earth.

It's the way to ensure you don't waste your one life but instead maintain a decluttered life—the life you've always wanted. It won't be perfect or problem free. But it will be lighter, freer, authentic, and finally focused on who and what matters.

Inner Decluttering Tool: Replace Conforming Habits

Spend time in prayer today. God waits for you in your inner home ("for he lives with you and will be in you"; John 14:17). Ask him to reveal habits in your life that you need to let go of because they're leading you away from him. Make a list of whatever comes up. Maybe it's listening to the news because it stirs up fear. Maybe it's scrolling Instagram before bed because it fosters anxiety and comparison. Maybe it's checking email immediately upon waking because the tone of your day is now set on earthly things.

What habits can you replace?

- Listen to a soul-filling podcast instead of the news.
- Read a spiritual book before bed instead of scrolling Instagram.
- Spend time in prayer and Scripture in the morning instead of checking email.

In *The Power of Habit*, author Charles Duhigg suggests that we can't end habits; we can only replace them. For habit replacing, he uses the model of cue, routine, reward. The habit you want to replace is your cue (grabbing for your phone to scroll social media before bed), the replacement behavior is the new routine (grabbing a great spiritual book instead), and the reward is the benefit that comes from the new routine (you feel more peaceful and less anxious before bed).

Commit to pushing back against one thing that's causing you to conform. Replace it with a habit that facilitates transformation. If you slip one day, simply start again the next. Ask the Holy Spirit to give you strength, and he will.

Outer Decluttering Tool: Tackle Daily Tasks

Choose two two-minute tasks from the daily maintenance task list:

- Make your bed.
- Place shoes in designated spots.

Do these two tasks daily for the next several days.

Once you have them down, add in a third task from the list.

- Recycle junk mail.

Do these three tasks for several days, then add in a fourth task.

- Empty full trash cans.

Continuing adding a new task every three to four days (be sure to delegate some to your spouse and kids). Soon these daily tasks will be second nature and your home will feel much less cluttered.

EYES ON HEAVEN

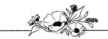

Aim at heaven and you will get earth
thrown in. Aim at earth and you get
neither.

—C. S. LEWIS

It's a Tuesday morning. My back rests against the recliner
chair—the same one I sat in at the start of my minimalism journey. I watch September rays illuminate my clear
surroundings.

I'm there, but not really. Intentionally this time, though.
My mind and my heart are lifted in prayer. The September
sunlight, the recliner, and the clutter-free bedroom quickly
coalesce, memories surface, and soon I'm thanking God for
the path that changed my life, the journey that freed me to
feel my soul again.

A creak from the bedroom door breaks my contempla-
tive state. My blonde-haired girl peeks in, her blue eyes wide,

expectant. She's far from the baby she was when I began my minimalist journey—she's six now. The days in our first rental home have passed, and, unshackled from consumer debt, our family of six now resides in a purposefully small new build. I meet Elena's unwavering gaze with an inviting smile. She enters and, after scanning for a seat, chooses my lap.

Five years have passed since I accepted my Spirit-led challenge to escape consumerism and realign my identity with God's. To live a life of meaning, a life without regrets. A life without excess inner and outer stuff.

I breathe in Elena's scent, which carries mischievous hints of chocolate. (It's only 7:00 a.m.) I tousle her unruly mass of bedhead. Would she still choose my lap if our lifestyle had never changed? A life numbed by clutter wasn't conducive to relationships. A life where the people around me were moving "to-dos" didn't foster connection or love. Would I have even begun to know her if I had never pursued simplicity? I glance at the Bible beside us. Would I have even begun to know God?

I think of the words of the apostle John: "By this we may know that we are in him: whoever says he abides in him ought to walk in the same way in which he walked" (1 John 2:5–6 ESV). By God's grace, I'd made the needed space to align the steps of my earthly journey more closely with his.

Elena slings her long legs over the armrest and flashes me a gap-toothed grin. As I think about my journey, I'm tempted to regret all the years I gave to physical and spiritual clutter—to conspicuous consumption, untrue inner narratives, distraction, and materialism. But my gratitude for a new life—a rich life—displaces any remorse.

♡

I wish I could tell you that my journey to amass the things that matter never has missteps. That I have this simplicity thing 100 percent down by now. That I never rush, never react, and never succumb to my "phone twitch loop." That I never feel the inner tug to buy myself or my children things as an attempt to boost happiness.

But I *can* tell you this: I'm different now. When consumerism whispers its empty promises and I listen, when my eyes shift downward to a screen, when I start to wonder what others might think, this clutter no longer has the upper hand. I can catch it now; I can observe it now. And just as quickly as it encroaches, I can let it go.

I now have the space, awareness, and tools to choose: live under the weight of the inner and outer clutter that stifles my soul, or excise it and free myself to connect with who and what matters.

I've chosen the latter. What will you choose?

Can you imagine yourself as the "living house" C. S. Lewis describes that "God comes in to rebuild"?[1] Do you feel his intent knocking, calling you to live differently? Feeling it is one thing. Answering it is another.

Choosing the path of physical and spiritual house-clearing isn't easy. It's not for the faint of heart. Because once you go all in, your very soul gets unearthed. Your facades drop, and you have nothing left to hide behind. In this raw, real exposure, your heart, mind, and soul become open, finally having the capacity to unite with God.

We're all on a path. A path that started when we entered the world empty handed and continues as we leave this world empty handed. We're given the freedom to choose what we do in between.

♡

Elena reaches a small, covertly-chocolate-tinged hand upward. It lands gently on my cheek and, after resting a moment, glides toward my chin. "What are you thinking about, Mama?" she murmurs. My eyes drift toward hers. "I'm thinking about what it means to be rich in what matters," I say.

She doesn't probe further, but if she asks for a fuller response someday, maybe when she's older, I'd simply answer this . . .

To be rich in what matters is to shift your focus from earthly treasures that are transient, fleeting, and ephemeral to eternal treasures that never perish or fade.

And when she's older, God willing, I'll still be here, eyes on heaven, in the world but increasingly not of it, continuing my journey down simplicity's path until it leads me to my forever home.

So here's to decluttering our hearts, minds, and souls and creating space to fill them with the things above.

Here's to letting go.

Here's to opting for the lighter yoke.

Here's to wanting the One who matters most—who is greater than any possession we could ever hold.

ACKNOWLEDGMENTS

My journey into simplicity hasn't been one I've walked alone. I'm deeply grateful for everyone who has joined me on this journey, has helped me see what really matters, and has been involved in the making of this book.

- Justin—Thanks for all the times you've said, "I think you should go for it." It's your support that made this book happen. I love you and love life with you.
- Eva, Elena, Ethan, Emelia, and Evelyn—You are our gifts. Thank you for filling my world with so much joy. I love you forever.
- Julia Kovac—I'm not sure this book would exist without you. Thanks for introducing me to minimalism and encouraging me to write. I've learned so much from you, and I am grateful.
- Julie Gwinn—Thanks for the out-of-the-blue Instagram message. I'm beyond thankful that you noticed my work and reached out. I'm grateful for your support through the entire book-writing process!
- Andrea Palpant Dilley—This book is immeasurably

better because of you. You are an expert at decluttering manuscripts. I'm grateful to have worked with you on this project!

- Kim Tanner—Your attention to detail and accuracy is unmatched. Thank you for your wonderful final edits that helped refine and improve this book!
- The Zondervan team—Thanks for all your time and dedication to this project. It's been an absolute joy to work with you all!
- My parents, Ann and Dan Nurse—You're the best. Your support means so much. I love you!
- David and Taylor Nurse, "my creative team"—Thanks for the brainstorming sessions and continued encouragement. Love you both!
- Paul and Rebecca Nurse and family—Thanks for your love and support!
- Ella McTavish—You're like family. Thanks for everything the past several years!
- Julie and Jeff Ubbenga—I'm grateful for your continued support and prayers!
- Beatriz Rodríguez-Rabadán—Happy to call you "sis"! Thanks for the love and prayers.
- Molly Price and Adrienne Doring—You were my cheerleaders during this book-writing process. Thanks! It meant a lot!
- To everyone who is part of the Rich In What Matters community—Thank you for all the blog posts you've read, kind comments and emails you've written, social media posts you've shared, and thoughtful DMs you've sent. I'm grateful for every one of you; this book is

because of you. I love community with you—less is truly more!

- God the Father, the Son, and the Holy Spirit—Love Infinite, Love Incarnate, Love Within. My gratitude to you goes beyond words. Simplicity has given me the space to know you. I'm forever grateful. You inspired me in the writing of this book, and all the good that comes from it is because of you! Thank you.

NOTES

Introduction

1. Peter Walsh, *It's All Too Much: An Easy Plan for Living a Richer Life with Less Stuff* (Los Angeles: Free Press, 2007).
2. C. S. Lewis, *Mere Christianity* (HarperCollins: New York, 2001), 205.
3. "Mother Teresa," Crossroads Initiative, accessed August 14, 2024, https://www.crossroadsinitiative.com/saints/quotes -from-blessed-mother-teresa-of-calcutta/.

Chapter 1: Stressed Out by Stuff

1. Margot Adler, "Behind the Ever-Expanding American Dream House," NPR, July 4, 2006, https://www.npr.org /templates/story/story.php?storyId=5525283.
2. Jack Feuer, "The Clutter Culture," *UCLA Magazine*, July 1, 2012, https://newsroom.ucla.edu/magazine/center-everyday -lives-families-suburban-america.
3. Harry Enten, "American Happiness Hits Record Lows," CNN, February 2, 2022, https://www.cnn.com/2022/02 /02/politics/unhappiness-americans-gallup-analysis/index .html.
4. Mary MacVean, "For Many People, Gathering Possessions Is Just the Stuff of Life," *Los Angeles Times*, March 21, 2014, https://www.latimes.com/health/la-xpm-2014-mar-21-la -he-keeping-stuff-20140322-story.html.
5. "Survey Finds 54 Percent of Americans Are Overwhelmed with Clutter and Don't Know What to Do With It," PR

Newswire, January 13, 2015, https://www.prnewswire.com /news-releases/survey-finds-54-percent-of-americans-are -overwhelmed-with-clutter-and-dont-know-what-to-do -with-it-300019518.html.

6. Joshua Fields Millburn, "Inside the Prison Walls of Consumerism," *The Minimalists* (blog), accessed February 28, 2023, https://www.theminimalists.com/prison/.

7. Feuer, "Clutter Culture."

8. Jeanne E. Arnold, Anthony P. Graesch, Enzo Ragazzini, Elinor Ochs, *Life at Home in the Twenty-first Century,* (Los Angeles: The Costen Institute of Archaeology Press, 2012), 28.

9. Feuer, "Clutter Culture."

10. Quoted in Feuer, "Clutter Culture."

11. Bishop Fulton Sheen (@Bishop_Sheen), "You must remember to love people and use things, rather than to love things and use people," Twitter, December 9, 2023, 11:52 a.m., https://twitter.com/Bishop_Sheen/status /1733530178830123098.

12. Brian Schieber, "The Road Map to Happiness," *Homily Podcast*, January 29, 2023, https://podcasts.apple.com/us /podcast/january-29-2023-the-road-map-to-happiness /id1558511182?i=1000597135292.

13. "Signature of Divine (Yahweh)," track 1 on NEEDTOBREATHE, *The Heat*, Atlantic/Lava, 2007.

14. Brian Schieber, "The Road Map to Happiness."

15. Louise Story, "Anywhere the Eye Can See, It's Likely to See an Ad," *New York Times*, January 15, 2007, https://www .nytimes.com/2007/01/15/business/media/15everywhere .html?pagewanted=all&_r=0.

Chapter 2: Minimalism: An Invitation to Freedom

1. Jan Johnson, *Abundant Simplicity: Discovering the Unhurried Rhythms of Grace* (Downers Grove, IL: InterVarsity Press, 2011).

2. Joshua Fields Millburn and Ryan Nicodemus, "What Is Minimalism?" *The Minimalists* (blog), accessed May 7, 2023, https://www.theminimalists.com/minimalism/.

3. Millburn and Nicodemus, "What Is Minimalism?"

4. John Mark Comer, *The Ruthless Elimination of Hurry* (Colorado Springs: WaterBrook, 2019), 76–77.

5. Josh Miller, "The Spirituality of Subtraction," *First15 Daily Devotional*, accessed February 28, 2023, https://www.first15.org/articles/the-spirituality-of-subtraction/.

6. Comer, *Ruthless Elimination of Hurry*, 201.

7. Mike Nudelman, Chris Weller, "9 of History's Greatest Philosophers Reveal the Secret to Happiness," *Independent*, January 12, 2017, https://www.independent.co.uk/life-style/philosophers-nietzsche-socrates-secret-to-happiness-a7524371.html.

8. Leo Babauta, *The Power of Less* (New York: Hachette, 2009), ix.

9. Joshua Becker, *The More of Less: Finding the Life You Want Under Everything You Own* (Colorado Springs: WaterBrook, 2016), 9.

10. This is my adaptation of Becker, *More of Less*, 8–11.

11. Becker, *More of Less*, 12.

12. Joshua Becker, *Things That Matter* (Colorado Springs: WaterBrook, 2022), 6.

Chapter 3: Redefining Rich: A Closer Look at Money

1. Alexandria White, "Americans Have an Average of 4 Credit Cards—Is That Too Many?" CNBC, May 10, 2022, updated July 25, 2024, https://www.cnbc.com/select/how-many-credit-cards-does-the-average-american-have/.

2. Jessica Dickler, "US Households Now Have over $16,000 in Credit-Card Debt," CNBC, December 13, 2016, https://www.cnbc.com/2016/12/13/us-households-now-have-over-16k-in-credit-card-debt.html.

3. Peter Stromberg, "Do Americans Consume Too Much?" *Psychology Today*, July 29, 2012, https://www.psychologytoday.com/intl/blog/sex-drugs-and-boredom/201207/do-americans-consume-too-much.
4. Joshua Fields Millburn and Ryan Nicodemus, *Love People, Use Things: Because the Opposite Never Works* (New York: Celadon, 2021), 188.
5. Aimee Picchi, "More than 60% of Americans Are Living Paycheck to Paycheck. Here's What Researchers Say Is to Blame," CBS News, August 31, 2023, https://www.cbsnews.com/news/paycheck-to-paycheck-6-in-10-americans-lendingclub/.
6. "Bible Verses about Money and Stewardship," Envoy Financial, accessed February 14, 2023, https://www.envoyfinancial.com/participantresources/bible-verses-about-money-and-stewardship.
7. C. S. Lewis, *Mere Christianity*, (HarperCollins: New York, 2001), 213–14.
8. Siddharth Vishwanathan, "Sadio Mane, Liverpool Star's Cracked iPhone Breaks Fans Hearts but His Response Is Legendary," News Nation, January 9, 2020, https://english.newsnationtv.com/sports/football/sadio-mane-cracked-iphone-liverpool-premier-league-250281.html.
9. Vishwanathan, "Sadio Mane, Liverpool Star's Cracked iPhone Breaks Fans Hearts but His Response Is Legendary."
10. Tristen K. Inagaki and Lauren P. Ross, "Neural Correlates of Giving Social Support: Differences between Giving and Targeted versus Untargeted Support," *Psychosomatic Medicine* 80, no. 8 (October 2018): 724–32, https://doi.org/10.1097/PSY.0000000000000623.
11. American Psychological Association, *Stress in America: Are Teens Adopting Adults' Stress Habits?*, February 11, 2014, https://www.apa.org/news/press/releases/stress/2013/stress-report.pdf.

12. "Two-Thirds of Americans Have Decreased Spending Due to Economy, Wells Fargo Money Study Finds," Wells Fargo, February 27, 2024, https://newsroom.wf.com/English /news-releases/news-release-details/2024/Two-thirds-of -Americans-have-decreased-spending-due-to-economy -Wells-Fargo-Money-Study-finds/default.aspx.

13. Max Roser, "The History of the End of Poverty Has Just Begun," Our World in Data, January 11, 2022, https:// ourworldindata.org/history-of-poverty-has-just-begun.

14. Cait Flanders, *The Year of Less* (Carlsbad, CA: Hay House, 2018), 162.

15. Cait Flanders, "You Weren't Born to Pay Off Debt and Die," *Huffington Post*, April 14, 2016, https://www.huffpost .com/archive/ca/entry/you-werent-born-to-pay-off-debt -and-die_b_9692684.

16. *The Minimalists: Less Is Now*, directed by Matt D'Avella, aired 2021 on Netflix, https://www.netflix.com/watch /81074662?source=35.

17. Faiza Malik et al., "Impact of Minimalist Practices on Consumer Happiness and Financial Well-Being," *Journal of Retailing and Consumer Services* 73 (January 2023), https:// doi.org/10.1016/j.jretconser.2023.103333.

18. Malik et al., "Impact of Minimalist Practices."

19. Jon Mooallem, "The Self-Storage Self," *New York Times Magazine*, September 2, 2009, https://www.nytimes.com /2009/09/06/magazine/06self-storage-t.html.

20. "Jerry Seinfeld on 'Tonight Show': Everything Becomes Garbage," Deadline, December 24, 2014, https://deadline .com/2014/12/jerry-seinfeld-tonight-show-garbage-video -1201335222/.

21. Elizabeth Siegel, "Can You Use Coconut Oil as Makeup Remover?" *Allure*, March 12, 2015, https://www.allure.com /story/coconut-oil-makeup-remover.

22. Ramit Sethi, "You've Got Money All Wrong: A Step by

Step Guide to Living a Rich Life," *The Mel Robbins Podcast*, April 26, 2023, https://podcasts.apple.com/us/podcast/youve-got-money-all-wrong-a-step-by-step-guide-to/id1646101002?i=1000610810165.

23. Sethi, "You've Got Money All Wrong."
24. Sethi, "You've Got Money All Wrong."
25. Sethi, "You've Got Money All Wrong."
26. C. S. Lewis, *The Problem of Pain* (San Francisco: HarperCollins, 1996), 106–7.

Chapter 4: Letting Go

1. Brooke McAlary, *Slow: Simple Living for a Frantic World* (Naperville: Sourcebooks, 2018), 8.
2. Brooke McAlary, "Exclusive: When Brooke McAlary Wrote Her Own Eulogy, She Had No Idea It Would Change Her Life Forever," Now to Love, January 5, 2022, https://www.nowtolove.com.au/news/real-life/i-wrote-my-own-euology-brooke-mcalary-70415.
3. McAlary, "Exclusive: When Brooke McAlary Wrote Her Own Eulogy, She Had No Idea It Would Change Her Life Forever."

Chapter 5: Awakening to the Spirit Within

1. Quoted in John Ortberg, *Soul Keeping* (Grand Rapids: Zondervan, 2014), 23.
2. Edward Ahn, "Jettison the Self-Propelled Motor and Be Wind-Powered," *Marian Priest* (podcast), May 28, 2023, https://podcasters.spotify.com/pod/show/edward-ahn9/episodes/JETTISON-the-self-propelled-motor—be-Wind-powered–Pentecost-Sunday-e24qede.
3. William Irvine, *A Guide to the Good Life: The Ancient Art of Stoic Joy* (New York: Oxford University Press, 2019), 1–2.
4. Myquillyn Smith, *Cozy Minimalist Home* (Grand Rapids, MI: Zondervan, 2018), 60.

5. Teresa of Avila, *The Interior Castle* (Charlotte: TAN Books, 2011), 7.
6. Carrie Gress, *Theology of Home: Finding the Eternal in the Everyday* (Charlotte, NC: TAN Books, 2019), 19.
7. Emily P. Freeman, "A Soul Minimalist's Guide to Letting Go," *Emily P. Freeman* (blog), accessed June 30, 2023, https://emilypfreeman.com/soul-minimalists-guide -letting-go.

Chapter 6: Inner Decluttering Challenges

1. Shira Gill, *Minimalista* (New York: Ten Speed Press, 2021), 15.
2. Joyce Meyer (@JoyceMeyer), "You cannot have a positive life and a negative mind," Twitter, June 18, 2023, 2:30 p.m., https://twitter.com/JoyceMeyer/status /1670499121868701696.
3. Daniel G. Amen, *Healing the Hardware of the Soul* (New York: Free Press, 2002), 160–70.
4. "How Many Thoughts Do We Have per Minute?" Reference, August 4, 2015, https://www.reference .com/science-technology/many-thoughts-per-minute -cb7fcf22ebbf8466.
5. Fran Simone, "Negative Self-Talk: Don't Let It Overwhelm You," *Psychology Today*, December 4, 2017, https://www .psychologytoday.com/us/blog/family-affair/201712 /negative-self-talk-dont-let-it-overwhelm-you.
6. R. B. Zajonc, "Attitudinal Effects of Mere Exposure," *Journal of Personality and Social Psychology* 9, no. 2 (1968): 1–27, https://doi.org/10.1037/h0025848.
7. Daniel Kahneman et al., "Anomalies: The Endowment Effect, Loss Aversion, and Status Quo Bias," *Journal of Economic Perspectives* 5, no. 1 (Winter 1991): 193–206, https://doi.org/10.1257/jep.5.1.193.

8. Kahneman et al., "Anomalies: The Endowment Effect," 193–206.
9. Marie Kondo, *The Life-Changing Magic of Tidying Up* (New York: Ten Speed Press, 2014), 60.
10. Courtney Carver, *Soulful Simplicity* (New York: TarcherPerigee, 2017), 53–55.
11. Carver, *Soulful Simplicity*, 55.
12. Joshua Fields Millburn, "Getting Rid of Just-in-Case Items: 20 Dollars, 20 Minutes," *The Minimalists* (blog), accessed August 6, 2024, https://www.theminimalists.com/jic/.
13. Quoted in Jostein Nielsen, ". . . Without Us God Will Not," Salvation Army, December 5, 2018, https://salvationarmyeet.org/without-us-god-will-not/.

Chapter 7: Outer Decluttering Challenges

1. "Ready to Spring Clean? The Cleaning Authority® Says Start by De-Cluttering," PR Newswire, March 20, 2015, https://www.prnewswire.com/news-releases/ready-to-spring-clean-the-cleaning-authority-says-start-by-de-cluttering-300053707.html.
2. Julia Stoll, "U.S. TV Consumption: Daily Viewing Time 2009–2023, By Age Group," Statistica, July 4, 2024, https://www.statista.com/statistics/411775/average-daily-time-watching-tv-us-by-age/.
3. Darby E. Saxbe and Rena Repetti, "No Place like Home: Home Tours Correlate with Daily Patterns of Mood and Cortisol," *Personality and Social Psychology Bulletin* 36, no. 1 (January 2010): 71–81, https://doi.org/10.1177/0146167209352864.
4. Emilie Le Beau Lucchesi, "The Unbearable Heaviness of Clutter," *New York Times*, January 3, 2019, https://www.nytimes.com/2019/01/03/well/mind/clutter-stress-procrastination-psychology.html.

5. Erica Layne, *The Minimalist Way* (San Antonio: Althea, 2019), 55.

6. Stephanie McMains and Sabine Kastner, "Interactions of Top-Down and Bottom-Up Mechanisms in Human Visual Cortex," *Journal of Neuroscience* 31, no. 2 (January 2011): 587–97, https://doi.org/10.1523/JNEUROSCI.3766-10 .2011.

7. Ann Voskamp, "Dear Me, Lines to the Person I Want to Be," *Ann Voskamp* (blog), July 6, 2022, https://annvoskamp .com/2022/07/dear-me-lines-to-the-person-i-want-to-be/.

Chapter 8: Decluttering the Kitchen and Letting Go of Restlessness

1. Gabrielle Bossis, *He and I* (Boston: Pauline Books & Media, 2013), 265.

2. Kevin Salwen, *The Power of Half: One Family's Decision to Stop Taking and Start Giving Back* (Boston: Mariner Books, 2011).

3. Francine Jay (@miss.minimalist), "My goal is not to get more done, but to have less to do," Instagram, March 18, 2019, https://www.instagram.com/p /BvJ5O5aB6Vq/?igsh=MXczYWo3dG5hcncyYg==.

4. Erin Keller, "Americans Spend More than 400 Hours a Year in the Kitchen: Poll," *New York Post*, August 3, 2022, https://nypost.com/2022/08/03/americans-spend-more -than-400-hours-a-year-in-the-kitchen-poll/.

5. "Exposure to Chemicals in Plastic," Breastcancer.org, October 12, 2023, https://www.breastcancer.org/risk/risk -factors/exposure-to-chemicals-in-plastic.

6. "A 1985 Newspaper Essay, Popularized on the Internet, Comes Full Circle," *L.A. Times*, November 22, 1998, https://www.latimes.com/archives/la-xpm-1998-nov-22-me -46549-story.html.

7. Jack Feuer, "The Clutter Culture," *UCLA Magazine*, July 1, 2012, https://newsroom.ucla.edu/magazine/center-everyday -lives-families-suburban-america.

8. Lisa Woodruff, *The Paper Solution: What to Shred, What to Save, and How to Stop It from Taking Over Your Life* (New York: G. P. Putnam's Sons, 2020).

9. Jacques Philippe, *Searching for and Maintaining Peace* (New York: Society of St. Paul, 2002), 5.

10. Richard Foster, *Prayer: Finding the Heart's True Home* (San Francisco: HarperOne, 2002).

Chapter 9: Decluttering Your Wardrobe and Letting Go of Comparison

1. Quoted in Jacques Philippe, *Searching for and Maintaining Peace* (New York: Society of St. Paul, 2002), 42.

2. Gabrielle Bossis, *He and I* (1948; Boston: Pauline Books & Media, 2013), 60.

3. Deborah Weinswig, "Millennials Go Minimal: The Decluttering Lifestyle Trend That Is Taking Over," *Forbes*, September 7, 2016, https://www.forbes.com/sites /deborahweinswig/2016/09/07/millennials-go-minimal-the -decluttering-lifestyle-trend-that-is-taking-over/.

4. Joan Kennedy, "The Life Cycle of a Viral Fashion Trend," *The Business of Fashion*, July 5, 2023, https://www .businessoffashion.com/articles/marketing-pr/the-life-cycle -of-a-viral-fashion-trend/.

5. Courtney Carver, *Project 333: The Minimalist Fashion Challenge That Proves Less Really Is So Much More* (New York: TarcherPerigee, 2020), 22–23.

6. "Universal Access to Safe Drinking Water Is a Fundamental Need and Human Right," UNICEF, July 2023, https://data .unicef.org/topic/water-and-sanitation/drinking-water/.

7. Jack Caporal, "American Households' Average Monthly Expenses: $6,081," *The Ascent*, December 1, 2023, updated

February 28, 2024, https://www.fool.com/the-ascent
/research/average-monthly-expenses/.

8. Olivia O'Bryon, "Pareto Is Perfecting the 20% of Clothing
Women Actually Wear," *Forbes*, May 1, 2022, https://
www.forbes.com/sites/oliviaobryon/2022/05/01/pareto-is
-perfecting-the-20-of-clothing-women-actually-wear/.

9. Zoya Gervis, "You're Not the Only One Who Constantly
Feels 'Wardrobe Panic,'" *New York Post*, March 7, 2018,
https://nypost.com/2018/03/07/youre-not-the-only-one
-who-constantly-feels-wardrobe-panic/.

10. Carver, *Project 333*, back cover.

11. Courtney Carver, *Soulful Simplicity, (New York:
TarcherPerigee, 2017)*, 95.

12. Cassandra Aarssen, *Real Life Organizing: Clean and Clutter-
Free in 15 Minutes a Day* (Miami: Mango, 2017), 98.

13. Mark Comer, *The Ruthless Elimination of Hurry*, (Colorado
Springs: WaterBrook, 2019), 248.

14. Joshua Fields Millburn and Ryan Nicodemus, *Essential:
Essays by The Minimalists* (Asymmetrical Press, 2015).

15. Carver, *Project 333*, 112.

16. Courtney Carver, "The Ultimate Guide on How to Start a
Capsule Wardrobe," Be More With Less, accessed May 25,
2024, https://bemorewithless.com/start-capsule-wardrobe/.

17. Joshua Becker, "Understanding the Diderot Effect Tto
Overcome Overspending," *Forbes*, October 27, 2021,
https://www.forbes.com/sites/joshuabecker/2021/10
/27/understanding-the-diderot-effect-to-overcome
-overspending/?sh=21b6cd3316fe.

18. Meghan L. Meyer and Matthew D. Lieberman, "Why
People Are Always Thinking about Themselves," *Journal
of Cognitive Neuroscience* 30, no. 5 (May 2018): 714–21,
https://doi.org/10.1162/jocn_a_01232.

19. John Tierney, "Do You Suffer from Decision Fatigue?"
New York Times Magazine, August 17, 2011, https://www

.nytimes.com/2011/08/21/magazine/do-you-suffer-from
-decision-fatigue.html.

20. "The Role of Gratitude in Spiritual Well-being in
Asymptomatic Heart Failure Patients," *Spirituality in Clinical
Practice* 2, no. 1 (March 2015): 5–17, https://doi.org/10.1037
/scp0000050.

Chapter 10: Decluttering the Living Room / Bedroom and Letting Go of Hurry

1. Mark Buchanan, *The Rest of God: Restoring Your Soul by
Resetting Your Sabbath* (Nashville: Nelson, 2007), 45.
2. Ann Voskamp, *One Thousand Gifts: A Dare to Live Fully
Right Where You Are* (Grand Rapids: Zondervan, 2010), 66.
3. Thomas Merton, *Conjectures of a Guilty Bystander*
(Doubleday Religion, 1968), 81.
4. Meyer Friedman and Ray H. Rosenman, *Type A Behavior
and Your Heart* (New York: Knopf, 1974), 42.
5. Josef Pieper, "Learning How to See Again," in *Only the
Lover Sings: Art and Contemplation* (San Francisco: Ignatius
Press, 1990), 33.
6. Pamela Todd, *William Morris and the Arts and Crafts Home*
(United Kingdom: Chronicle Books, 2005), 46.
7. Kimberly Horton, "The Effect Your Paint Color Has on
Your Mental and Physical Well Being," May 15, 2012,
https://designsbykh.com/color-psychology-effects-on
-humans/.
8. "Reading 'Can Help Reduce Stress,'" *Telegraph*, March 30,
2009, https://www.telegraph.co.uk/news/health/news
/5070874/Reading-can-help-reduce-stress.html.
9. Francine Jay, *The Joy of Less, A Minimalist Living Guide:
How to Declutter, Organize, and Simplify Your Life* (San
Francisco: Chronicle Books, 2016).
10. Quoted in Connie Whitman, "Improve Your Life by
Cleaning Out a Closet," Web Talk Radio, accessed August

13, 2024, https://webtalkradio.net/internet-talk-radio/2018
/06/25/improve-your-life-by-cleaning-out-a-closet/.

11. Lysa TerKeurst (@lysaterkeurst), "Whenever you say 'yes' to
    something, there is less of you for something else. Make sure
    your 'yes' is worth the less," Facebook, October 4, 2016,
    https://www.facebook.com/OfficialLysa/posts/whenever
    -you-say-yes-to-something-there-is-less-of-you-for
    -something-else-make-s/10153858105412694/.

12. Greg McKeown, *Essentialism: The Disciplined Pursuit of Less*
    (New York: Crown, 2014), 137.

13. "Diaphragmatic Breathing for GI Patients," University of
    Michigan Health, accessed July 25, 2024, https://www
    .uofmhealth.org/conditions-treatments/digestive-and-liver
    -health/diaphragmatic-breathing-gi-patients.

14. Brené Brown (@BreneBrown), "It takes courage to say yes
    to rest and play in a culture where exhaustion is seen as
    a status symbol," Twitter, July 21, 2021, https://x.com
    /BreneBrown/status/1417969468031045639.

Chapter 11: Decluttering Kids' Stuff and Letting Go of Reactivity

1. Josh Sanburn, "America's Clutter Problem," *Time*,
   March 12, 2015, https://time.com/3741849/americas
   -clutter-problem/.

2. Juliet B. Schor, *Born to Buy: The Commercialized Child and
   the New Consumer Culture* (New York: Scribner, 2004), 19.

3. Kim John Payne, with Lisa M. Ross, *Simplicity Parenting:
   Using the Extraordinary Power of Less to Raise Calmer,
   Happier, and More Secure Kids* (New York: Ballantine,
   2010), 59.

4. Payne, *Simplicity Parenting*, 65.

5. Payne, *Simplicity Parenting*, 65.

6. Quoted in Lori Rothstein and Denise Stromme, "Space
   between Stimulus and Response," University of Minnesota

Extension, March 2, 2021, https://extension.umn.edu/two
-you-video-series/space-between-stimulus-and-response.

7. Senay Canikli Adıgüzel et al., "The Effect of Cold
Application to the Lateral Neck Area on Peripheral
Vascular Access Pain: A Randomised Controlled Study,"
Journal of Clinical Medicine 12, no. 19 (October 2023):
6273, https://doi.org/10.3390/jcm12196273.

8. Martin Taylor, "Adult Coloring Books: 7 Benefits of
Coloring," WebMD, August 11, 2021, https://www.webmd
.com/balance/features/benefits-coloring-adults.

9. Jessica Migala, "7 Ways to Stimulate Your Vagus Nerve and
Why It Matters," Everyday Health, December 27, 2023,
https://www.everydayhealth.com/neurology/ways-to
-stimulate-your-vagus-nerve-and-why-it-matters/.

10. Payne, *Simplicity Parenting*, 62.

Chapter 12: Decluttering Sentimental Items and Letting Go of Fear

1. Katherine Weber, "Rick Warren: Why God Encourages
Christians to 'Fear Not' 365 Times in the Bible," *Christian
Post*, April 30, 2016, https://www.christianpost.com/news
/rick-warren-why-god-encourages-christians-to-fear-not
-365-times-in-the-bible.html.

2. Rosie Leizrowice, "The Psychology Of Sentimental Items
And How To Let Go Of Them," *Huffington Post*, March 17,
2018, https://www.huffingtonpost.co.uk/rosie-leizrowice
/the-psychology-of-sentime_b_15397710.html.

3. Marie Kondo, *The Life-Changing Magic of Tidying Up* (New
York: Ten Speed Press), 116–118.

4. Joshua Fields Millburn and Ryan Nicodemus, "The
Spontaneous Combustion Rule," *The Minimalists Podcast*,
YouTube, November 2, 2021, https://www.youtube.com
/watch?v=eOfApYEP4f0.

5. Patrick Lencioni, "If Everything Is Important...," The Table

Group, accessed July 30, 2024, https://www.tablegroup
.com/if-everything-is-important/.

6. Jacques Philippe, *Searching for and Maintaining Peace* (New York: Society of St. Paul, 2002), 26.

7. Philippe, *Searching for and Maintaining Peace*, 28.

8. Hillsong United, "Oceans (Where Feet May Fail)," Zion, August 23, 2013.

Chapter 13: Decluttering Your Digital World and Letting Go of Distraction

1. Rachel Macy Stafford, *Hands Free Mama: A Guide to Putting Down the Phone, Burning the To-Do List, and Letting Go of Perfection to Grasp What Really Matters!* (Grand Rapids: Zondervan, 2013), 219–20.

2. Alexus Bazen, "Cell Phone Statistics 2024," ConsumerAffairs.com, December 12, 2023, https://www .consumeraffairs.com/cell_phones/cell-phone-statistics.html.

3. Cal Newport, *Digital Minimalism: Choosing a Focused Life in a Noisy World* (New York: Portfolio/Penguin, 2019), xi.

4. Anna Lembke, *Dopamine Nation: Finding Balance in the Age of Indulgence* (New York: Dutton, 2021), 1.

5. Justin Worland, "How Your Cell Phone Distracts You Even When You're Not Using It," *Time*, December 4, 2014, https://time.com/3616383/cell-phone-distraction/.

6. Jonathan Haidt, *The Anxious Generation: How the Great Rewiring of Childhood Is Causing an Epidemic of Mental Illness* (New York: Penguin, 2024), 209.

7. Haidt, *Anxious Generation*, 208.

8. Haidt, *Anxious Generation*, 209.

9. Newport, *Digital Minimalism*, 28.

10. Alane K. Daugherty, "The Science of Novelty," *Psychology Today*, January 21, 2022, https://www.psychologytoday .com/us/blog/healing-stress-the-inside-out/202201/the -science-novelty.

11. Kent C. Berridge and Terry E. Robinson, "Liking, Wanting, and the Incentive-Sensitization Theory of Addiction," *American Psychologist* 71, no. 8 (November 2016): 670–79, https://doi.org/10.1037/amp0000059.
12. Marysia Weber, *Screen Addiction: Why You Can't Put That Phone Down* (St. Louis: En Route Books & Media, 2019).
13. Newport, *Digital Minimalism*, 109.
14. Mel Robbins (@melrobbins), "Don't miss out on your life because you're too busy scrolling through someone else's," Twitter, November 28, 2017, 10:08 p.m., https://twitter.com/melrobbins/status/935706886560800773.

Chapter 14: Maintenance Decluttering

1. Gabrielle Bossis, *He and I* (Boston: Pauline Books & Media, 2013), 247.
2. Rachelle Crawford (@abundantlifewithless), "Minimalism doesn't mean always tidy. It just means easily tidied," Instagram, May 20, 2022, https://www.instagram.com/p/Cdx4ROfAWlP/.
3. Flannery O'Connor, *The Habit of Being: Letters of Flannery O'Connor*, ed. Sally Fitzgerald (New York: Vintage, 1980), 229.
4. John Mark Comer, *Practicing the Way: Be with Jesus. Become like Him. Do as He Did.* (Colorado Springs: WaterBrook, 2024), 101.
5. Marie Kondo, *The Life-Changing Magic of Tidying Up,* (New York: Ten Speed Press, 2014), 142.
6. David Nurse, *Pivot and Go: The 29-Day Blueprint to Redefine and Achieve YOUR Success* (Herndon, VA: Amplify Publishing, 2020), 49–52.
7. Joshua Fields Millburn and Ryan Nicodemus, *Love People, Use Things: Because the Opposite Never Works* (New York: Celadon, 2021), 62–65.
8. Millburn, *Love People, Use Things*, 63.

9. Millburn, *Love People, Use Things*, 64.

10. Millburn, *Love People, Use Things*, 53.

11. Darrell Stetler II, "21 Times Jesus Said 'Follow Me,'" Newstart Discipleship, March 20, 2024, https://www .newstartdiscipleship.com/post/21-times-jesus-said-follow -me.

12. Comer, *Practicing the Way*, 181–92.

13. Comer, *Practicing the Way*, 192.

14. Comer, *Practicing the Way*, 99.

15. Comer, *Practicing the Way*, 177.

Epilogue: Eyes on Heaven

1. C. S. Lewis, *Mere Christianity*, (HarperCollins: New York, 2001), 205.

From the Publisher

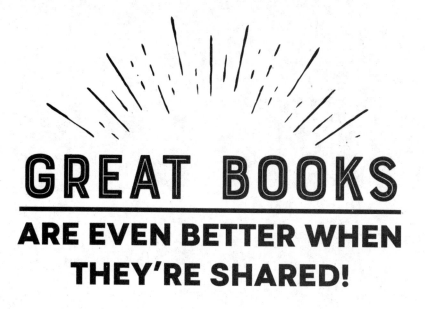

GREAT BOOKS
ARE EVEN BETTER WHEN THEY'RE SHARED!

Help other readers find this one:

- Post a review at your favorite online bookseller

- Post a picture on a social media account and share why you enjoyed it

- Send a note to a friend who would also love it—or better yet, give them a copy

Thanks for reading!